Caring for Madness
The role of personal experience in the training of mental health nurses

To Pa, who was always concerned about my education

Caring for Madness
The role of personal experience in the training of mental health nurses

Seevalingum Ramsamy

PhD, BEd(Hons), MEd, PGCE, CERT Ed, RNT, DNPsych, RMN, RGN, Department of Mental Health and Learning Disability, Sheffield University

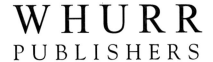

WHURR
PUBLISHERS

© 2001 Whurr Publishers Ltd
First published 2001 by
Whurr Publishers Ltd
19b Compton Terrace
London N1 2UN England, and 325 Chestnut Street, Philadelphia
PA 19106, USA

Reprinted 2003

British Library Cataloguing in Publication Data
A catalogue record for this book is available from the British
Library.

ISBN 186156 200 4

£ 25 - 29

Printed and bound in the UK by Athenaeum Press Ltd,
Gateshead, Tyne & Wear

Contents

Foreword

This is a significant book in a number of respects. In the first place, there are relatively few accounts of the experiences of nurses in training. This neglect is, perhaps, not surprising when one considers that research in nurse education is still largely influenced by quantitative methodologies, in which the student voice is not heard, but such approaches are particularly inappropriate in inquiries into the training of psychiatric nurses given the nature of their role. Such nurses must necessarily draw upon their own personal resources – their experiences of coping with the trials and tribulations of life – if they are to deal effectively with the problems of patients, which are, by their very nature, expressed within a social context. If the training of these nurses is to be successful, it must clearly develop students' personal competencies, but it can only do this, one imagines, if it is based upon a knowledge of 'where the students are' in their own personal understanding. And, as George Kelly said many years ago (Kelly 1955), if you don't know what lies in your subjects' minds, you should ask them to tell you. This simple but often neglected advice is seriously followed in the present book, which provides many fascinating insights into students' perspectives as they are initiated into the profession.

This achievement alone makes this work essential reading for nurse educators and students alike, but what gives it added value is that the author places students' accounts within an historical framework. In the first part of the book, he shows how concepts of madness and caring for madness have evolved over the past three thousand years. We see that the use of models from the natural world in forming our ideas of cleansing the mind/body in mental illness has a long history and, arguably, extends inappropriately to the present day. On the other hand, there is from very early times evidence of the recognition of the importance of personal insight and development for both carer and cared-for in the treatment of mental illness. These different, often contradictory, emphases are of course still pervasive and help to determine the incoherent way in which the role of the psychiatric nurse is defined in practice.

For Dr Ramsamy, the way forward is to develop a philosophy of personal knowledge that can help us to integrate the personal and impersonal aspects of psychiatric nursing. Such a philosophy, he claims, will do justice to the interpersonal context of the nurse-client relationship, and it can form the basis for a curriculum for psychiatric nurse education. In the final section of his book, he draws upon the thoughts of authors such as Polanyi and Macmurray to outline his suggestions. These considerations are, I believe, vital if the curriculum offered to trainee psychiatric nurses is to be derived from considered judgements made in the light of theoretical understanding and research evidence. This book does not provide a ready-made curriculum. Its importance lies in its directing us to ask the right questions about the nature of training for psychiatric nurses.

Neil Bolton

Glossary

CFP	Common Foundation Programme
CPN	Community Psychiatric Nurse
ENB	English National Board
MDT	Multi-disciplinary Team
RCN	Royal College of Nursing
RMN	Registered Mental Nurse
RMPA	Registered Member of the Psychological Association
SEN	State Enrolled Nurse
UKCC	United Kingdom Central Council for Nursing, Midwifery and Health Visiting

Acknowledgements

I would like to give my particular thanks to Professor Neil Bolton, who encouraged me to undertake this study and guided me with imagination, patience and affection during the early stage of this thesis. Without his love and support, phenemonology would have been an impossible task. A special thanks to my supervisor Dr Peter Clough for his support.

I am grateful to the students who devoted their time to this research, and to Chris Lavender for her patience in typing my handwriting in readable words. I would also like to thank Nat, Palmeshiven, Kristopher, Di and my parents, Vadarajoo and Lorgambal Ramsamy.

'You would not find out the limits of the psyche, even though you should travel every road: so deep a logos does it have'.

Heraclitus

Chapter 1

Introduction

> Our experiences are ignored, we are made to feel as
> though we do not know what we are on about once we
> start psychiatric nurse training.
> Self-direction is an excuse for tutors not preparing
> lectures.
> It is a do-it-yourself course.

The form of the text

The above are representative of the types of statement from students
who urged me to undertake this project, which addresses the issue of
how personal experience can be used in the training of mental health
nurses. This project started from a practical base in the sense that information was collected before any theoretical ideas relating to the
personal experience of training were collected.

Thus, Section I comprises an historical account of notions of
madness and of caring for madness to show how the experience of
madness formed, at least in 'prescientific' times, a basis for the management of madness. Particular attention is paid to experiencing madness
in relation to the role of the 'attendant' of the asylum, this section
providing the foundation for applying a conceptual framework for
understanding the students' lived experiences. This is obvious in
Section II, where the methodology and style of research with regard to
the reported experiences of students has been described without my
trying to impose any prior theoretical framework. This section presents
students' own accounts of their experiences in training for psychiatric
nursing and is centrally concerned with how successfully students can
integrate personal experience into theoretical and institutional
formats. The categorizing of the student data is based upon the integration of protocols guided by the prior historical analysis.

In the final section, I turn to relevant philosophical and educational literature concerned with the development of reflective practice and student autonomy. I suggest a framework for developing the effective usage of student experiences in psychiatric nurse training, which will, hopefully, prove helpful to programme-planners.

Section I consists of two parts. The first deals with the Vedic culture, Egyptian times and the Greek perspective. These three approaches form the bedrock for the management of madness. In fact, through reading the first section, it becomes obvious that the ideology behind the techniques used in the management of madness today was in place during the Vedic and Egyptian times. The Greeks in turn inherited and systematized the ideas of these different cultures, the approach that they proposed still being followed in a number of respects. There are many similarities between these early concepts of madness and its treatment and more recent approaches allegedly based upon a scientific perspective, that is, those taken from nineteenth-century accounts. There are a number of existing reports of the history of the concept of madness and the development of the lunatic asylum (see, for example, Foucault 1961; Scull 1962; Porter 1985), which start from the time of the Enlightenment with an outline of the Greek system. I have of course borrowed from these, but I have also taken the historical perspective further back in time to include early Asian, Egyptian and Greek viewpoints. In so doing, the similarities between the early conceptualization of care and the allegedly scientific accounts of the Enlightenment and the nineteenth century become obvious. This thesis goes beyond the Socratic time and describes how the Socratic approach was influenced by early cultures.

The second part of the historical section outlines the management of madness through the Enlightenment, with its emphasis on such practices as blood-letting, purging, beating, electrocution, flooding and incarceration, to chemical chaining – the use of chemical tranquillizers as a form of harnessing madness.

In Section II, as I indicated earlier, students undergoing training gave their accounts of experiencing the course. It was intended that students be given as much freedom as possible in producing these accounts. In Chapter 7, data from individual accounts are reported, and Chapter 8 consists of a commentary of group discussions and clinical experiences during training.

In categorizing these responses, the historical analysis is used to show the major themes. There is therefore a continuity between past and present-day concerns in the care of madness. This style of relationship between history and the presentation of students' lived experiences is a new approach, as will become obvious in the beginning of Section III.

Section III deals with the future of mental health nursing from the point of view of personal experience, attempting to integrate historical perspectives with the students' experiences of training and recent research relevant to mental health nursing. The research targets the use of experience in the training of preregistration mental health students.

Having presented this critique, Section III goes on to outline a philosophy for mental health nursing based on the use of personal knowledge and a form of experiential learning. This perspective builds upon accounts, the comments made by several of the students who perceived their training to be a form of personal development rather than just specific training for a task. The purpose of elaborating the main features of this mental health mode is to put forward a model for a developmental process for reflective practice.

Although this thesis draws students from two different syllabuses, the 1982 syllabus and Project 2000, my purpose is not to point out any difference that this produces. This work is instead concerned essentially with the relevance of experience to the training of mental health nurses and should not be seen as an evaluation of these two curricula.

The philosophical perspective of the thesis

This text is informed by a phenomenological perspective, not in the sense of following a phenomenological method for understanding social or psychological events, but in terms of its adoption of the philosophy of existential phenomenology. This philosophy is made explicit in Section III but has also been influential in Section I, as well as in Section II, which attempts, through eliciting students' views of their experiences in training, to illuminate their lived experience.

Against Husserl's (1969) attempt to find a pure, transcendental phenomenology of experience, Heidegger (1978) argued that our starting point must be the everyday world, that 'everydayness' in which one is caught up in an absorption in ordinary affairs. The first goal of understanding is to capture the way in which we encounter things in the everyday world without our explicitly noticing their nature (p. 79).

Heidegger's phenomenology of human agency starts out from a description of life as a happening, caught up in its dealing in ordinary contexts. We shall in this thesis, for example, see that, in this context, the students relied upon and used their mentors, the patients, the clinical staff, the teaching staff, their lived experiences and their personal networks. All these are ready to hand, the material around which students can organize their understanding of the nature and aim of caring, and ultimately 'round up' their interpretations as agents in this world. These contexts gain their significance not only from the interactions that necessarily occur, but also from the actions of the agents defining the context. We shall see that students' descriptions of their experiences in the workshops bring out the ways in which their lives are always nested in the wider contexts of a historically generated culture.

The possibility of self-interpretation and particular ways of acting is generally guided in advance by public role standards and conventions. From this perspective, individuals are primarily participants and place-holders in what Heidegger (1978) calls the *Dasein* or existence. This attunement to public ways of acting, the ingrained tendency to respond according to social standards, is a primordial phenomenon that belongs to *Dasein*. What is being done at any time has a point and makes sense only against the backdrop of relevant practices and institutions. The completeness of situations within the world is where things matter to us because of our prior attunement. This aspect displays itself, as we shall see, in the students' accounts. As agents, we are outside ourselves in addressing the concerns of daily life; this is according to our cultural sense of what is important in dealing with objects and equipment.

But existential phenomenology never describes merely for the pleasure of describing. Ricoeur (1977) points out the examples of Hegel, Kierkegaard and Nietzsche, for whom description is effective only in the service of a great plan: to denounce an alienation, to rediscover the place of man in the world or to recover his metaphysical dimension.

What is pivotal in Heidegger's existential analysis of *Being and Time* (although, it must be said, neglected by the phenomenology character-istically adopted into the social sciences) is the distinction between authentic and inauthentic existence. Heidegger discovers three aspects or moments that are basic to the way in which *Dasein* 'stands in' the world. Each is a mode of *Dasein*'s standing-in, that is, of his freely relating himself to things. Consequently, each is open to the possible variation that freedom introduces.

Dasein, in projecting the fundamental acts of standing-in, can in the case of each of the three modes do so either authentically or inauthen-tically. An authentic mode of standing-in is based on *Dasein*'s relating itself to things in view of the whole structure of what it really is. An inauthentic mode finds *Dasein* so concerned with the necessities of daily life that it relates itself to things by projections that ignore the implications of the full structure of its possibilities. For each authentic mode of comportment towards the things that are, discovery of self as already in the world (*Befindlichkeit*), understanding (*Verstehen*) and discourse (*Rede*), there exists a corresponding inauthentic form: ambiguity (*Zweideutigkeit*), curiosity (*Neugier*) and prattle (*Gerede*).

Each mode is only one aspect of standing-in and hence is always to be found with the others. For example, understanding *Dasein*'s central way of existing would be impossible without that basic presence to the things-that-are, natural to *Dasein* from birth. Similarly, there would be no such *Befindlichkeit* if it were not the very essence of *Dasein* to stand in the world by interpreting or understanding. Nor would there be an understanding were there no expression of what is understood. Expression being the function of discourse, it follows that *Rede* is the essential fulfilment of *Verstehen*.

From this analysis of the authentic modes of *Dasein*'s being-in-the-world, we can conclude that the basic concern of *Dasein* is an involvement in things-of-an-intentional-kind understanding. This self-assertion among the things-that-are is supposed to be at once docile, drawing its substance from things as they are, and creative, bringing the illumination of meaning to things in the act of discourse. The authentic act of standing-in is an act of existence involving a self-extension toward what is unknown and is not yet, so that meaning may be brought to be and new explanations offered for the things-that-are. Authentic existence is poetic in nature. Poetry, as Heidegger conceives it, is respectful of things, respectful of the meanings created by past generations as an expression of the correct possibilities of those epochs, while remaining conscious of its responsibility as creator of new meaning in casting original light on the things-that-are.

The possibilities of inauthenticity are not mere negations of the authentic modes; they are as much positive, concrete realities of *Dasein* as the authentic. Ontologically, both are on the same footing, and both always go together to form the two faces of finitude, somewhat as act and potency always go together in the Aristotelian conception of the finite thing. As a result of *Dasein*'s finitude, he is thrown into a world dominated by concern for the necessities of survival. Heidegger speaks of this condition of the 'everyday *Dasein*' as his *Verfallensein*, which he seeks to express as a positive phenomenon. This not-being-itself functions as a positive possibility of *Dasein*, resulting from the *Dasein*'s concerned involvement in the world.

We should understand that we are encountering here the reality of *Dasein*'s essential finitude. Because it is finite, the *Dasein* never achieves a pure revelation of Being in a perfect relationship to the things-that-are, untrammeled by narrow considerations. Each revelation, each 'interpretation', is partial; consequently, its very affirmations must exclude. Authentic existence can only be something of an ideal, a direction to aim at amidst the dark reality of the dissimulation of everyday life.

The *Dasein* of the average man becomes so involved in the necessary search for bread and in the concern for what 'they' say that it ignores the reality of his own existence. The authentic existent, however, is ready to sacrifice all to the service of the creative renewing powers of his own poetic nature. The effort to surpass metaphysics, to which Heidegger's philosophy is devoted, should be viewed in the existential perspective of 'Sein and Zeit'. The forgetting of being that has characterized the Western tradition is the counterpart on the level of philosophical criticism of the Verfallensein on the level of the concrete existential act. The surpassing of this tradition is the act required of the authentic Dasein, which would review an awareness of the holiness of Ek-sistenz, or authenticity.

Heidegger terms the kind of involvement that characterizes the Dasein of the daily world a 'Zweideutigkeit'. The curious phenomenon signified by the term is that the man who is caught up in the whirlpool of daily activity is the least straightforward in his dealing with things. Dasein gets so involved in 'going along with the crowd' that he can soon no longer distinguish their catchwords and pat formula answers from what is revealed in pure understanding.

This proves something about the very nature of the act of understanding, namely that it does not function in a vacuum of pure reason but is fundamentally based on the projections that underlie my way of relating myself to the world. The ambiguity arises from the interplay of conflicting elements in my interpretation: the influences of the echte Verstehen and the point of view and presuppositions I bring to the thing. The average Dasein's involvement in things, once infected with ambiguity, lacks the foundation to achieve anything but a superficial handling of reality.

The second mode of standing-in becomes, in the fallen state, curiosity instead of genuine understanding. Curiosity, which often passes in the world as a virtue and sounds so original, is in its superficiality interested only in uncovering what is trite and can never invent new horizons of its own. 'He is interested in seeing, but only in seeing', says Heidegger (1978), 'and not in understanding, that is to say in ein Sein zu ihm zu kommen'.

The expression of the curious Dasein is prattle (Gerede), the inauthentic counterpart of discourse. Prattle dramatizes the doubtful nature of inauthentic existence. It serves as a positive block to genuine discourse, the clanging noise that drives away the great silence indispensable for the kind of discourse that touches the essence of things.

The significance of Heidegger's analysis of authentic and inauthentic existence for this thesis is to prepare us to see the student experience of learning to care in terms of both the necessary context provided by established social structures and perspectives and the choices made by students as they attempt to make sense of what they do to arrive at morally justified actions. In Section III, I propose a moral-developmental approach to reflective practice that is, I believe, appropriate for the caring professions.

The text begins with an examination of the history of madness and of caring for madness. It does so not in the belief that history determines absolutely our present behaviour, but in the same way that Heidegger (1968) and Merleau-Ponty (1962) have argued for the continuity of the past with the present. Heidegger (1978) makes the point that finding myself among the things-that-are and coming to realize that their presence before me depends on my opening a horizon of interpretation (*Verstehen*) and that I actively let the objective thing be through the discourse (*Rede*) that is the outcome of my acts of interpretation.

The source of each of the three modes is thus traced directly to my own finite reality and the unity of the three is discovered to be rooted in my finite existence. I come to see that every movement of authentic existence must unite care for each of the *Ektases* or frenzies, the past, the present and the future: the past that I must actively assimilate as part of an authentic *Befindlichkeit*, the future that I build out through the projections of *Verstehen*, and the present of that dwelling with the things-that-are that takes place in the *Rede*, which expresses my grasp of things.

The past reveals itself to me in terms of human possibility and my projections, that is, what I count possible, and determines what I shall objectively 'see' or overlook. The *Dasein* that does not shoulder the burden of his destiny (*Schicksal*), either because he ignores the past or because he ignores his responsibility towards the future, becomes the tool of fate and blind arbitrariness, both of which are only aspects of his own inauthenticity. *Wiederholung* and *Uberlieferung* are the names that Heidegger gives to the two aspects of *Dasein*'s authentic historical development. Repetition, the act of making present the possibilities of the past in view of his resolute projections, is the basis of 'handing on a tradition', which is what occurs when I actualise historical possibility on the basis of what has been done and thus make possible new advances for the future.

History, in Heidegger's view, is above all the other sciences concerned with the concrete. He argues that in no other science is the 'generally valid' a less possible criterion of truth than in authentic history. How then can historical research be said to have scientific value? If history has to do neither with the facts, which being purely concrete can have no applicability elsewhere, nor with general laws that would abstract from the concreteness of existence to the point that it loses its validity, history's scientific value depends on a new kind of applicability. This is the existential applicability in which the theme of history is concerned neither with that which happens only once, nor with some generality that hovers over the facts, but with the factually existent past possibility. Such possibility can never be repeated, that is, historically understood authentically, as long as it is turned into the paleness of a super-temporal model. Only factually authentic historicity as resolute destiny can so reveal past history that in repeating our history we will enact and fulfil our own possibilities.

It is in this spirit of analysis of the significance of history that Section I offers an historical account of the development of caring for madness.

Section I

An Historical Approach to the Management of Madness

Chapter 2
Historical background

The management of madness has, historically, been associated with different concepts of human nature since madness is defined as some sort of failure of that nature. Necessarily, therefore, in this first section I shall be concerned with the way in which different cultures have conceptualized madness in relation to different philosophies of life and how this has informed the task of caring for madness. In fact, we shall see considerable continuity from Vedic to recent times.

The historical account will show that the elements that constitute the self and madness are: the physical being, the environment, the ethical dimension, the education process and the divine power or science. These five poles identified by the history of human nature still play a great part in the process of caring for the self and madness. What has happened during the advancement of time is that these five forms have been refined by our knowledge and experience, leaving the principle behind the management slightly altered. Tracing from the Vedic time of India and through Egyptian and Greek history, we can see a similarity in their approaches in that they viewed the world in positive and negative forms, the process of being in the world being a friction between these two forces. This account will follow this principle, looking at how the self was perceived and how madness was viewed and managed through historical development.

The historical section will be presented in two parts. Chapter 3 will offer summary accounts of three early civilizations. The first is that of the Vedic time, which is the South Indian history rooted in a culture that predated the history of ancient India, 2468BC, by 500 years (Wheelan 1961, 230). The term used to describe this ancient philosophical psychology is Sanatana Dharma (Nathan 1983, 8). The Egyptian time was traced to a beginning at about 3200BC (Alfred 1961). The section on the Egyptian account perceived the Nile to be the essence of life, the place where the seeds of Western civilisation was sown in the Valley of the Nile (Alfred 1961, p99). The third culture is that of Ancient Greece, placed from around 3000BC (Hood 1961, 195–228).

By exposing these three ancient cultures, I will show the view of the self, the ethics of the times and the perception and management of madness. This will be followed by a summary. The continuity and contradiction in these different perspectives will be drawn together at the end of this section.

This historical account will describe the continuity and similarities between the cultures and will also confirm how this ancient knowledge still has an impact on the present principles of care. The institutionalization of madness – the birth of the asylum – was a gathering not only of the mad, but also of the carers, the lunatic attendants. The attendants were an element of control, but they found themselves also being controlled by this process of incarceration.

Chapter 4 covers madness and caring for madness from the Enlightenment to the present time, providing an account of the recent history of psychiatry and the role of attendants/mental health nurses over this period. The question that will be raised at this point is how the mechanical form of restraint came to overrule the developmental approach to care from the Enlightenment onwards.

Chapter 3

Madness and views of the self in early civilization

This part describes the self and the management of madness, taking into account the ethical aspects of self and care. It will cover:

- Vedic time;
- Egyptian history;
- Ancient Greek civilization.

The Vedic tradition

The ancient culture of Asia is used to include the three traditions of Charvaka, Buddhism and Jainism (Chinmayananda 1979, 11). The Charvaka were those who believed in self-indulgence, sensuousness and living from day to day. The Buddhists revolted against the Vedic ritual, denied eternal existence and saw life as an ever-changing series of acts of consciousness, flickering in the intelligence, whereas Jainism denied the Vedanta but believed in eternal truth.

The Vedantic tradition was not bound down by rigid commandments, orders, declarations and revelations; it was passed by word of mouth through generations. It was this style that allowed the sapling an unrestricted growth. Like the Banyan tree, it gave birth to different branches that developed adventitious roots, as there are branches, to anchor it in the soil (Chinmayananda 1983, 20). Each branch helps the mother tree in its search for sustenance, as well as being self-maintained. As a unit, it forms part of the beauty of the forest, acting as support and shelter for nature and its entities. It is the symbol of the tradition, and, like any symbol, it has a form, a bark, to hold it in place.

Before dissecting the Vedic tradition, we have to know the structure and how the different parts are placed in the Gestalt. We have to perceive the whole as it is the whole that is made up of the parts, and it is

13

the way and process of putting them together again that makes the sum bigger than the whole.

This style is that of the fluidity of the Vedanta in that there are different versions of the Veda, the Reg Veda being the form that holds and supports the others (Chinmayananda 1979). It is this style of inter-relatedness, with a structure arranged in a traditional way, that makes the Veda's storage of scientific knowledge the soil of the Vedic culture. The tradition addresses itself to the soil, the elements of nature. In the process of self-confrontation during meditation, this Gestalt has to be taken into account. The Vedic literature prescribed the scientific method of how to reflect and confront one's experiences, but, because of its fluidity, it did not provide definite conclusions.

Nature and ethics

Nature is arranged in an ethical way. What makes it ethical is that god is found in every object, subject and interactive process (Aiyar 1983, 33–47). Thoughts, words, language are the sounds of the gods (Brahman), which manifest themselves in different ways (Aiyar 1983, 39). In the same way in which the divine departments control nature, they also control the seen and unseen aspects of the human experience. Offerings, ceremonial activities and sacrifices, in the form of feasting and taking part in processions, are ways of compensating the gods (Nathan 1983, 57–63; 335–6). Not carrying out a religious promise or ritual may lead to disaster or illness.

The ethical is part of our action in dealing with nature, people or things. Action that involves non-action and not doing what one should do is acting in an irresponsible way. The basic rules of action (according to Reede 1983, 29) are:

- *Ahimsa* – non-harming and non-hurting, which refers to pain of any physical nature;
- *Virtue* – the true source in emotional life, which involves;
- *Asteya* – intention, as it is the faculty or the self that guides our actions and, importantly, openness in action.

How we act towards others forms our embodied experience, Vasanas, (Chinmayananda 1979); this experience and the awareness of it form part of consciousness. In the Indian culture, the third eye (consciousness) is the spot between the eyebrows, the Commanding Wheel, its freedom being declared by its decoration with the Sacred Ash, Vibhuti, the silver ashes to which the body turns. Vibhuti is the symbolic form of Krishna, the positive, and Shiva, the negative. These are the two charges or opposites that Vishnu used to produce language by means of the Conch (Nathan 1983, 65–72; see also Chinmayananda 1979, 331–4, vol 1). Although the third eye accepts the finite, it is infinite and indestructible, being in reincarnation our Vasanas, which has to occupy another space to give itself a form to confront itself.

The power of the ashes, as indicated, and the infinity of consciousness are what form the power of sound, knowledge and language. Knowledge here forms part of consciousness as the third eye, which passes on to another body or vehicle. It is also embodied in the vehicle, the body, which when rendered to ashes becomes the form of language. This is an indication that dualism is not only the domain of the age of reason, that is, the seventeenth century. There is a two-fold system in the Vasanas: experience, like language, has both negative and positive aspects (Akhilananda 1951, 20–3).

It is this infinity of consciousness, the power to transcend and confront, that is being in the world. Our action is exhausted through confrontation with the world, so that consciousness is both in the world and always seeking to move beyond it. We have already seen that transcendence is embodied in our knowledge, language and action (Vasanas); this is the whole foundation on which our freedom is based, as will be discussed later. In the above description, I have pointed out that Sanatana Dharma presents a natural and holistic approach in that nature (our environment) is inseparable from us even in death. Now it is time to show the disembodiment of this human self.

The dissected self

The self is seen as splitting itself into two divisions. First, it keeps close to nature and the social situation, and second, when the structure of human need is examined, it is found to occur not in a hierarchical style, as presented by Maslow (1968), but as a system threaded with needs at different stages running into each other. The two-fold nature of the self, together with its ethical development, including our embodied experience, goes to form the aspect of the self, or self-development.

In the first division, the place of nature and the environment is of great significance, in that the shadow provided by a group of trees growing harmoniously is of great symbolic power, especially if they are of an odd number with one opening from the soil. The forest, the rivers and the wilderness are the laboratory in which mediation and reflection are possible. The geographical position, or environment, is one aspect that describes our being; those from the east of the country look coarse and hard because of the climate and type of seasonal variation. The margose, which is a bitter vegetable, can only be eaten by a certain type of person, the black coarse-skinned mountain people (Chinmayananda 1978, 136). Regime and environment influence our state of being, our emotional profile, our intellectual stature and the imprint of life's experiences.

The first aspect of the psychology of being is made up of three parts, all embodied in every one of us (Chinmayananda 1978, 136–8). These three qualities – the Sattwic, the Rajastic and the Tamasic – give rise to a fourth one, the Sudras:

1. *Sattwic.* This is the temperament of the Brahman (this term referring to the ideal of knowledge and self-power, not to be confused with the distortion of it, Brahman, the high caste, which only flourishes through distortion and opportunism). It is that part of us which is curious, scientific and exploratory. Those who develop this quality are highly sensitive and peaceful.
2. *Rajastic/Tamasic.* This human quality is of two stages (the second and third), depending on the situation: there are the dynamic type – the politicians, those who act – and the traders and commercially minded.
3. *Sudras.* This is the muscular aspect of the self that carries out our intentions, political thoughts and material desires. This quality is what society oppresses and delegates to the 'workers'.

How we develop any one, or a mixture, of these aspects depends on where we are situated at birth and how we are cared for. However, the four qualities and how we develop them do not rest only on the accident of our birth, but also on how we organize ourselves and the nature of work undertaken.

The aim of the swami in encouraging self-development is to help to exhaust their own particular interest. Then, when the strength of one's qualities are rediscovered, the healthy mind should be uncluttered and individuals will have a clear vision with which to apprehend and modulate their relationship within the world (Chinmayananda 1978, 139–40; 173).

Second is personality structure, which was originally described in the *Taittiriya Upanishand*. The Food Sheath is composed of the five elements of the universe – earth, water, fire, air and the faculty of insight. It is the physical body, encompassing all our bodily systems, and is the way by which the ego gains experience and acts as the instrument for carrying out its mission. What gives the different parts their power is the deities presiding over them. The organs work in co-ordination to allow the body to act (Chinmayananda 1974, 8; 1979, 132).

The vital Air Sheath is the life energy, the physiological function (Chinmayananda 1979, 138–44). It is the power that presides over our creativity and the nucleus of all energy in ourselves.

The Mental Sheath is the sector of doubts, joys and similar emotions (Chinmayananda 1979, 145–51). It constantly erupts into the non-stop flow of the lava of thought. It is the 'Ganges', an incessant flow of thoughts directed towards certain destinations. This flow is the mind that creates its own power from the source of experiences and through the sense organs, the priests firing it with fuel (information). The mind is kept alight, not only from sensations and experiences, but also as a result of its own power blazing from its historicity, of which it may not be fully aware. The mind is not as a reflection of oneself in a mirror, in that it throws back what it senses, but the subject, enjoyer of objects and the creator of itself.

The next sheath, the Intellectual Sheath, is what the Rishi, the author of *Taittiriya Upanishad*, perceives as the human form, with faith as its head (Chinmayananda 1979, 149–50). The Vedanta describes it as having a head, faith and two sides. Ritman, the right side, comprises the textbooks we have to digest and what propels us to knowledge, Satyam, the courage of conviction, being the left side. The body is Yoga, the power that joins our life, imperfect or perfect being, to the attunement of self, the 'Truth' and the power in oneself. Yoga is self-refinement from different levels of the self-unfolding of spirituality (meditation).

The head, faith itself, is courage, the ability to grasp ourselves and have confidence in what we are doing. Faith is the sacred, most important limb without which we cannot leap into our future plane; without it, we become limp. Faith, courage and knowledge, when harnessed, constitute the power of truth, which gives us confidence and assertion. One who has lost confidence in himself is a lunatic, a danger to himself and society.

The Vedanta projects us as growing from intellect, study and training in the walk of life. The Yoga, the body of knowledge, has to refine itself in an ethical form, through meditation, the cutting edge of reflection, in order to consolidate and transcend the trunk of power. Transcendence is the power, the force and the confidence to move through one's situation in life, and being prepared through faith in one's action to move in the different levels of our situation.

In Vedantic literature, intellect is the mind that has come to a decision or a willed judgement. The intellect is the characteristic of the agent that controls perception. In the process of doing so, the agent 'I' undergoes a change in action – I develop awareness, which fuels my experience. In order to exhaust my experience, I have to move from one field of experience to another, so there are births and deaths, again and again (Chinmayananda 1979; Taittiriya Upanishand). The body, the sense organs, experience and my own embodiment constitute the 'I' that is consciousness. Consciousness is constantly singing its breathless duet as it constitutes an unbroken experience and the doubt of our decision in lived experiences. Being aware of consciousness playing upon the mind, the intellect and the ego is what illuminates the self.

Consciousness is the infinite power, the 'I-ness', which transcends the body. The knowledge of one's experience is what sacrifices itself for consciousness. Knowledge is Brahman and reflection, the sacrifice of Brahman being the ethic in action. A consciousness of something is what can cripple us to a state of madness or disintegration. We shall consider this point later.

The intellect is the supporting pivot of the Bliss Sheath (Chinmayananda 1979, 153–4). It is all the flickering joys that we encounter in the finite world of matter, as when the sense organs inhabit them. This virile soul also has a human form – joy is the head, rejoicing the left side, happiness the right side, bliss the trunk and Brahman the knowledge, with a supporting tail.

Joy derives from our experiences, both from our finite aspect of sense experience and the place we occupy, and from the infinity of conscious-ness, the power of the third eye, the universality and historicity of being. It is mental brooding, a contemplation of our wish or love object, the kind of mood, smile or any style of revealing ourself, that we cannot explain. The nearness of the love object and our wish is a delightful and enjoyable vicinity. This closeness makes joy subtler, rejoicing and happi-ness being the actual indulgence in the enjoyment of the object of expectation. Bliss is a stage of self-realization. The nearness of our expectation is not all happiness and calmness: it is also the power that can choke an agitated mind. Our level of self-realization is sorrow or the absence of it. Real joy is Brahman (Chinmayananda 1979, 159).

Brahman is knowledge, and knowledge is a form of Vasanas (experi-ence). It was pointed out that our experience is finite and infinite, and that our experiences are grounded in nature and ethics. Nature, as an environment guarded by the gods, is the space for meditation and creativity. Ethic is the respect in the way in which we interact with nature, how we interact with others and how our body itself interacts at a biological level.

This 'deified pan-ethico consciousness' penetrates every crease, crevice and sinus of the universe, just as the scientific gaze came after the dethronement of god. As described above, it is the consciousness and awareness of our experience that directs our actions, action being directed at the moment of intent: intention is action. The folding or unfolding of the self is the third aspect that harnesses the self.

The ethical, the harnessing of the self, is an infinite process of burning through our experiences (Akhilananda 1951, 11–23; Chinmayananda 1979, 25–58). Ethic is the fluid binding that holds the fragments of our Gestalt. To reach the ethical level of self-development is a tiresome and painful task of faith, an infinite involvement, a process of ongoing refinement in action.

Yama, self-development, is ethical and mental control. How this is achieved is not precisely prescribed, but the *Upanishad* laid down some rules to be enforced during action or interaction with others. Chief among these are principles to do with mental control. It is argued that the process of change is not repression but reprocessing and confronting ourselves to reach a level of self-realization. (Indian philosophy considers the unconscious to be a source of energy that holds our culture and historicity, as well as to be the fountain of creativity.) Change is seen as redirecting. In the process of redirecting, we should see ourselves as being in the world; self-detachment is being part of the world.

Being in the world allows me the freedom to move and act. My freedom within the situation entails obeying the rules and respecting others, as our actions will influence each other. Being an individual in the world allows me a space between 'I' and the others; in my moment of tension and anxiety, I can reflect on my actions without pouring them on the whole situation. Self-detachment is a kind of bracketing of one's personal experience in dealing with others. To self-detach is to be in, without allowing oneself to be overcome by, the whole situation. In the state of self-detachment, we can perceive what is threatening us in the situation of our daily activity and our own fragmentation or anxieties.

To be part of a situation is to see ourselves as a notch in a chain of events: any action influences us. If we allow our own personal experience to fragment over the situation, this leads to confusion and conflict in that we cannot differentiate between what is happening to us and to others. This situation thus depowers us, in that the tension within us and around us is so high that the flow of our experiences and skills in dealing with the situation is blocked, our whole being becoming fragmented. In that kind of situation, the mouth is parched, the body shivers all over, with sweat pouring, the skin begins to burn, the mind is whirling and the whole embodiment slips. The self has lost its power to aim and to direct its intention towards the focal point. Allowing oneself to be a vagrant in the chain of events is madness. In that situation, we need a mentor's ear and a sense of redirection; this is what the Bhagavad-Gita prescribes.

The mentors are those who are in a superior position, masters in the arena of their specific field of experience (Bhaktivedanta & Prabhupanda 1986, 81, 92–3, 103, 581). They may agree to be friends, sons or lovers, but they are still the masters. In being friends with their students, they do not assume being at the same level as instruction at this level is meaningless and deluded by illusionary energy. Students who have forgotten themselves in these situations are the forgotten souls, deluded by illusion. The mentors are those who openly accept the mastery of their skills and direct their students in how to listen to themselves and others.

Mentors are those who have followed the rules, regulations and principles in order to rise up to the platform of knowledge, and it is these facets which they display that liberate us from the clutches of delusion. Violence as a way of getting the instruction through is permitted, reflection being the most violent form in redirecting a student. The form of behaviour that the mentors display is what directs and facilitates the students. It is accepting one's position as a mentor, being respectful to the naivety of the students and being prepared to show one's form as a mentor, which may be termed a 'transcendental caring reciprocation' between students and mentor.

Silence and meditation are what forms the trunk of the Mental Sheath and the Intellectual Sheath. Reflection is mental cleansing. Physical cleanliness involves dietetic restriction and self-devotion. Madness is the involvement of oneself in a situation without sufficient self-direction: it is a disability that cripples our consciousness. The possible way out of this disability is to be directed by a mentor who will take us back to the crossroads at which we can rediscover our direction.

Perception of madness

The Vedic viewed madness as being possession by god, as in the case of chronic illness. The body itself was guarded by deities, but any weakness would lead to illness. This could be cured by fasting, sacrifice, meditation and religious activities. Internal conflict and not having the confidence to apply oneself to a situation was seen as a kind of weakness that cripples the self. Madness was also described as a vagrancy in the blood. The Vedic identified three humours responsible for madness and diseases of the body. The Rig Veda recommended meditation and prayers to the gods to keep the humours at bay. Water was perceived as the virile medicine and the dissipator of disease. Plant juices mixed with ghee, butter, lard or barley were the form of body purification (Ayyar & Giriza 1957).

Summary

In this perspective, human 'being' is seen as part of nature. Our actions and surroundings are controlled by the gods and by knowledge. How we present ourselves defines our position. We all have the potential to become a swami, a politician, a merchant or a manual labourer. How we develop ourselves in becoming a member of these groups depends on our determination, our developmental process and where we are placed at birth. The development of the self is also portrayed as self-realization. The Vedanta describes the physical body as the vehicle that fuels the self. Here we see that there is a gap between the physical body and the self. This dualism of the body and the self is, however, not absolutely clear, as knowledge of the self is embedded in the physical body, the ashes that decorate the eye of consciousness.

The self in its dissected form does not consist of hierarchical levels, for the different aspects support and fuel each other. Although each part is presented as a trunk of complete form, the parts depend on and support each other in a kind of symbiotic relationship. What goes to form the self are our Vasanas and our experience. Experience and consciousness are both finite and infinite, our culture and historicity being part of our make-up. Our relationships with others are controlled by ethics and self-discipline. Self-detachment is not withdrawal for it involves showing respect, care, understanding and being in the situation; it is caring for oneself and others.

Being involved in and preoccupied with a chain of events that is not directly related to what we are doing, especially if the involvement is personal and emotional, is what cripples our whole intention. What redirects us out of this crisis is the ear of the mentor. This will involve giving time, listening to what we have to say, clarifying some of our concerns, re-arming ourselves with ideas, even if it means reminding us of our situation. When Arjunar the warrior was crippled with the anxiety and dread at fighting during the Mahabarata, the great war, it was his mentor, Krishna, who redirected him towards his target (Chinmayananda 1978). This description of the self and madness occurred at the time of the Vedanta (650BC). The self has been presented as part of nature and under the gaze of the deity.

The fasting, offerings, sacrifices and promises to the gods were part of the process of cure and meditation. Sacrifice, the offering of animal blood to the gods after one has recovered from an illness or succeeded in one's project, has always been part of the Vedic form, although this does not mean that bleeding has always been symbolic. Blood was also under attack as a source of madness in the Vedic time; apart from purging the blood by means of herbs and fasting, bleeding was also prescribed to drive out one of the three humours.

The history of madness, like madness itself, is fragmented. The Vedic account is not a continuous flow, nor does it flow from Vedic time into Greek and Roman eras, its development being scattered all over history. The blood as a target in the treatment of madness is evident in the Vedic times but the approach was also influenced by the natural surroundings. The Egyptians, like the ancient Indians, attached meaning to the rivers and to their surroundings.

The Egyptian view of madness and the self

The Egyptian history of the self arose from African influences that saw madness as the state of being possessed by the spirits of the dead, but one of its major preoccupations was the model it took of human nature from the influence of the Nile (Thorwald, 1962, 16–19, 26, Note 39; Ellenberger 1974, 3–27). The Nile was described as the cradle of culture and what happened to and around the Nile as the model for illness of the human body.

The river's strength and range during certain seasons could not be controlled by the divine power of the king, Zoser, who had to appeal directly to other gods for help. The power of the Nile could strip the king of his godhead; during the dry season, it could kill most of the population by malaria and water-borne diseases. At this time, the black mark lining left behind (as an alluvial deposit) by the recession of the water became the source of economic power when cultivated, and a source of madness when ingested or injected by nature (similar to the malaria injected by mosquitoes). The Nile took a human form in ancient Egypt.

By the year 450BC, Egyptian medicine started separating medical practice into specialist branches, and diseases were seen in terms of organic lesions (Thorwald 1962, 41, 43). The Egyptians described diseases as an extensive hardening of the arteries and fat deposits caused by an overindulgence in food and drink. The Nile and its waters were the source of death in the lower classes, the river itself being divided in an anatomical way to represent her power in medical history.

The Egyptians developed their ideas of physiology and pathology through reason and through observing their surroundings. To achieve this end, they gathered information from observing dissections during the embalming of bodies and also from the slaughtered bodies of sacrificial animals supplied to them.

They did not want to follow the dull acceptance that physiology and pathology were controlled by the gods, wanting instead to build a system of knowledge based on anatomy and physiology. They saw diseases as being associated with organs with a hollow space in the middle, for example the abdominal organs (Thorwald 1962, 40, 76).

As a model of human physiology, the Egyptians were also attracted by the way in which the channels they dug controlled the flow of water from the Nile. To them, there must have been a similar system in operation controlling the flow of body fluids by the pumping power of the heart. The human body thus came to be structured on the model of the Nile and its channels, which carried the stream of water, the harnesser of the rage of the Nile, feeding different lakes. This was in turn used to provide water to mould the dry, baked soil to form the wet, dry, moist, warm medium seen as providing the roots with minerals, the organic bricks of human beings (Thorwald 1962, 75–6).

The channels leaving the heart (36 in all) were found to have a content similar to that of the fluid of the Nile in that they carried both nourishment and disease (Thorwald 1962, 76). They were to carry air, blood, mucus, nourishment, semen, excreta and the constituent of the black bile that resulted in madness and delirious behaviour. These channels were also responsible for inflammation, fever and other illnesses (Thorwald 1962, 88–9). They were to be kept clear from any slight blockage that might have interfered with the distribution of water. Just as a failure of the Nile, in that too high or too low a flow crest would block the smooth irrigation canals and destroy the land, so any alteration in the irrigation of the bodily system would be the cause of bodily disorders (Kaplan & Sadock 1985, 25–77).

Not only was the overflow or low level of fluid seen to be the source of madness, but it was also the elements that the fluid carried, as well as the blockage, that led to stagnation and disease. This takes us back to the belly and lining of the Nile, the black deposit lining the river, the endometrium responsible for protecting and feeding the seed during its developmental stage. This black lining was the source of richness when the Nile dried up during drought or water recession, the plantation flourishing and the fertility of the people along its valley increasing. When the lining was water-logged and blocked with river weed and other forms of grass, it became a source of madness in which the germs of insanity were hoarded; during plantation this would be transmitted to the food chain and the environment to become the humour in the black bile, the source of madness.

To treat the situation, the small streams left during the receding of the water were linked together to form deep rivers, thus creating a smoothly flowing stream. Weeds and grass were cut down and set on fire, smoking the germs away. (These two forms of managing the Nile were to play havoc in the treatment of madness and of female sexuality in relationship to madness.) The practices of cutting the vegetation Nile, smoking the crevices and scraping the mud were to become the management of madness.

The Hellenic Egyptian taxonomy of phlebotomy of the Nile, to remove the black humour, was to dominate madness until the late nineteenth century. But has it now disappeared? The circulatory system is still under attack, dementia being believed to result from a failure of the blood circulation. The low level, the drought season, in depression and schizophrenia is seen as being caused by the low level of body enzymes. What is under question is still the humour.

We do not, however, perform phlebotomy or anastomosis to increase or decrease the flow of these enzymes. Instead, we now have the monoamine oxidase inhibitors and other groups of antidepressants that increase the flow of these bodily humours (enzymes) or dam them to cure depression. When the flow is too slow, in desperate situations, a current – electroconvulsive therapy – is used to stimulate and increase the flow of these brain humours.

Even though this form of attack on the blood has changed, the principle that madness is related to body fluid (the blood and its genetic form) and the environment, as well as the natural approach, is still with us. We do not use cattle horns or prongs to clear the source of madness, the natural approach the Egyptians used (Thorwald 1962, 77). Instead, we have moved to chemical design in that we now use lithium carbonate to displace the potassium ions in cases of manic depressive disorder (Kaplan & Sadock 1985, 47–55).

The Egyptians did not stop at cattle horns and prongs to get at the rage of madness, nor was phlebotomy the only tool against the black bile (Thorwald 1962, 78). Leeches and blood-sucking worms were also a prescribed form of management, as were body massage and herbal remedies (Thorwald 1962, 57, 79).

Thus it was that the beginning of the scientific approach to madness became associated with intervention on the human body. The body organs were measured and the action of the pulse recorded; it was data from recording and measurement that gave human beings power over themselves, removing it from the gods.

This move, however, was clearly associated with the need for surgery and dissection; just as the weeds along the Nile were cut and burned, surgery was performed to control madness. The head was to be shaved to let out the heat generated by the brain. As the small streams of the Nile during the drought were linked together by digging and cutting, so too could the human body be cured of madness. The skull was drilled to remove foreign particles and relieve pressure (Thorwald 1962, 158–9).

The drilling of the skull and the dissection of the brain by the scalpel were to undergo further refinement by the first half of the twentieth century and are still the recommended form of management for some severe psychiatric disorders. With the use of medical physics, X-ray machines and accurate measurement of where the cut should be made, madness can be carved by a nuclear implant that can dissect the diseased or disordered part, without affecting the remaining part of the brain. The operation of stereotactic thalmolectomy can now be performed after medical specialists have been consulted, and with the consent of the patient. Once the living clay has been dissected, it has to relearn life skills with the help of physiotherapy, speech therapy, nursing and social therapy; we now have an army of specialists to do this. Madness is, from this perspective, not only an abnormality in the elements that can be treated with chemically designed medication: the diseased part can be carved out too.

Our inheritance from the Valley of the Nile, as far as remoulding is concerned, did not stop with the brain, the area of psychosurgery. By that time, the medical gaze had moved to the depth of the belly of the Nile, the black bile, and had travelled the circulatory system, showing up every blockage, inflammation and abnormal humour. Now the practitioner's regard moved from the Nile as a focus to the environment of the Nile. There too the same principles were to be applied to sexuality in what may be described as a sociomedical approach to care.

In the same way as the cutting of the Nile was seasonal, phlebectomy was to be performed seasonally after the astrologist had been consulted and the cosmos of the patient mapped out (Thorwald 1962, 150–2). The methods used by the Egyptians were to be followed by Napier and others up until the end of the nineteenth century (MacDonald 1981, 8). Bleeding in winter was against medical practice as it weakened the patient.

The problem of syphilis was the major social concern of the Egyptian, and the Nile taxonomy as it applied to madness was also adopted and extensively developed by the Greeks and Romans. This involved circumcision of the male and female sexual organs (Thorwald 1962, 53). There is no evidence of major surgical removal of the vagina, labia, vulva and clitoris in the Egyptian era, as their belief was that the body should be kept intact after death so that the soul could later reinhabit it.

The pubic and axillary hair were to be shaved, just as the Nile was treated in Ancient Greek times during their occupation of Egypt (Simon, 1978, 246). The uterus was held to be a dangerous place, a place of disease, a source of madness itself, a place wherein arise 'humours, brackish, nitrous, boracious, acrid, mordant, shooting and bitterly tickling' (Simon 1978, 260). The uterus was believed to be guilty of causing suicide because of madness in the sickness of the virgin (Simon 1978, 258). The medical discourse to taint the uterus with the humour of the black bile of the Nile had started, a diagnosis that proved particularly longlasting.

The castigation of this body organ by surgery had to occur to ensure that there was no risk of infection during intercourse, or when diagnosing and curing the womb. Just as Empedocles banished disease around the river by means of fire and smoke, the same principle was applied to women with vaginal discharge. Squatting over smoking leaves in order to allow the smoke to rise up the 'flue' was the prescription. The burning of bracken and the cutting down of the weed were to appear again in the Middle Ages, when women who were suspected of being witches, or of being mad, had to parade in front of the judges with their skirts up and their pubic hair shaved, so that the court could check for any sign of the devil. Vaginal discharge was considered to be an indication of witchcraft or madness (Ackernecht 1968, 16).

The Nile was to teach us more about how different social classes were to be treated. The Babylonian priestesses, daughters of the royal families, were the only group of women who could be at the disposal of the priests of the temple of Ishtar (Thorwald 1962, 163). Intercourse with them was claimed to be a sacred art of rejuvenation. The royal priestesses, who sanctified physical love in every possible form, had no hindrance in getting married. Prostituting herself at the Ishtar temple door step was a sacrifice that every woman had to perform. The priestesses were left untouched and were not operated on, and it was only those who stayed in the temple permanently who were sterilized. As the servants of the gods, they could not be seen to be performing the act of creation.

The situation differed for other women: a woman who crushed the testicle of a man would have her nipple cut off. If she crushed a second testicle during a scuffle, both nipples were to be removed (Thorwald 1962, 163). The treatment of class differential had already penetrated the management of people.

The principle of unblocking the Nile to allow free flow was to be reawakened in the Hippocratic era and during the time of Harvey, who described the heart as a powerful pumping machine. Hippocrates makes the uterus all important in that every condition – respiratory difficulty, pressure in the loin, headache, drowsiness, toothache and even the sacred disease, epilepsy – was considered to arise from it (Simon 1978, 242).

These illnesses were particularly to be found in women not involved in sexual intercourse, the theory being that the dry, deprived uterus rises in search of moisture (like the black bile, the endometrium of the Nile, rises when it is dry). Retention of the menses resulted in a similar situation – loss of voice, coldness, palpitations and toothache. The treatment consisted of bandaging to prevent movement, wine taken orally, nose fumigation to repel the ascending uterus and aromatic fumigations inserted into the vagina to attract the uterus to its rightful place (Simon 1978, 243). Marriage, intercourse and procreation were prescribed for virgins or widows.

Pathology of the hymen and its consequences for the virgin were held to cause suicide, delusional ideas, raving madness, hanging and drowning. There was believed to be a blockage that stopped the blood from flowing. This retention of menstrual blood pressed on the diaphragm and heart, thereby caused mental symptoms. The treatment was removal of the blockage in the case of a virgin, or in the case of a married woman pregnancy to prevent relapse.

Harvey (see Hunter & MacAlpine 1963), a physician in the eighteenth century, was to revive the treatment. He prescribed 'poking' for any phlegmatic virgin in her late teens and of a middle-class background. Later on, Kraepelin (see Barham 1984) was to diagnose any middle-class women who were promiscuous as suffering from simple schizophrenia.

The hymen, the structure tainted with envy and the sin of masturbation, the organ that makes consciousness a subject and the actress an object of pleasure in the act, was to be targeted. This mesh, which can sanctify a social contract of marriage and, in some societies' view, give the woman her pride, was the obstructive cause of madness.

The practice of using perfume to keep the uterus in place has not shifted, but perfumed tampons for providing women with a feeling of security during menstruation have led to a number of deaths from toxic shock syndrome. Different forms of plug have been invented, some even with wings to give more confidence. Ethics is being ignored in the act of selling perfume to keep the uterus at bay, and all for the benefit of the materialists.

Besides the black bile and the blockage in the circulation leading to madness, the Nile was also associated with herbal remedies. Herbal medications were traded internationally with Asia and the Far East (Thorwald 1962, 69). In what we would consider a modern approach, the effect of the drugs on the brain was recorded, and the prescribed drug was weighed out rather than given haphazardly (Thorwald 1962, 63).

Summary

Egyptian beliefs, with their African influences, touched on the Indian approach at different points, in that Asia provided the herbal medicine. The orifices were still the sites and gates of the gods, and the excretions were the form of evil power. Sewage pharmacology was used in both cultures to treat illness and to keep away devils (Thorwald 1962, 63).

The domestic water system, sewage pipes, baths and steam baths were to be found in both parts of the world (Thorwald 1962, 192–3).

The Egyptians, however, moved to another level and started the dethronement of the gods and the beginning of science, not being content to leave things in the hands of the deities. They appointed a minister for the water system, with hygiene conditions attached – hands were to be washed before and after meals, the sexual organs were to be washed after intercourse, and anyone who had been in touch with a diseased person should not be approached as the person might be carrying the disease. They were well aware of the danger of cross-infection.

The self was seen as being of both the body and the soul. Death was the parting of the soul, a point where the two cultures touched (Mishima 1962). The difference is that the Vedic culture perceived the soul to be part of the body and consciousness as experience that transcended time and took on another form to exhaust itself. The Egyptians held the view that the mummified, derelict corpse should be kept, with all the necessary utensils, for the soul to occupy the body at a later date. Indian culture did not leave the corpse intact as they believed in transmigration of the soul, that is, that what one became depended on one's experience in this life.

Thus it was that an approach to the human body and self developed in line with the natural model provided by the behaviour of the Nile. The body was to be carved, measured and harnessed by pharmacology to control the passion and rage of the blood, the liquid soul that hoarded madness (Barker 1929, 4). The crises surrounding the Nile fostered a kind of knowledge based on what can be seen and measured, and this cemented being into nature. The body and how it was treated and structured was a mirror image of the Nile. Nature meant the environment, the body, what was eaten and interacted with. This line of approach was to be taken up in Hellenic medicine (Hunter & MacAlpine 1963, 431–3; Lethrer 1989, 552–3).

Apart from the different techniques that we inherited from the emphasis on the Nile, as mentioned above, we also received from the Egyptians the imprint of science based on sensory perception. They stated that, if you want to know people, you should watch how they behave in their environment and how their environment is structured. It was the external world that provided a model (the taxonomy of the Nile) for organizing the inner structure of the human being. This structure was what gave form to the content of Egyptian knowledge and to behaviour, and by altering the structure, the contextual form was altered, this in turn altering the behaviour. Treatment is based, therefore, on the principle of alteration of both physical organs and the environment. These changes will then affect the behaviour of human beings.

The Greek perspective

The Greeks also placed great emphasis on the interrelatedness of the environment and life forms. To Hippocrates and Galen, the two poles of life were the organism and the environment. The organism could in fact be understood in terms of what it ingested from nature. Diseases were seen as being of digestive origin, of involving what the organism took from the environment (Jones 1946, 5). Like the Egyptians, the Greeks saw food as consisting of humours. The era of Hippocrates and Galen was a synthesis of the pre-Socratic time, and they were to influence the history of medicine profoundly (Armand & Maurer 1982, 3–21).

The historical account will start from the time of Homer, who gave us a poetic representation of the human psyche. It is the form that the self took in Homeric poetry that Socrates described whilst propounding the rules for establishing the process of education in the republic. It was the content of Homer's writing that became an important source of psychoanalysis in this century, and his terminology still reigns over the psychodynamic approach to care.

Pythagoras was possibly the first to describe the form of the self. He argued that most things concerning human beings came in pairs of opposing elements and that opposites were the first principles of existence (Jones 1946, 3–4). Aetius, the compiler to Alcmaeon, believed that health was the balance and maintenance of equality among the powers and that diseases occurred as a result of one of the forces being autocratic (Hawkes 1980, 2). The humoural approach was to take the view that disease was caused by this autocracy or by an imbalance in one of the humours.

This section will describe the following:

- the Greek version of the self;
- the importance attached to the environment in Greek medicine;
- the ethics of the self;
- the Greek perspective on madness.

The self

The Indo-Europeans, ancestors of the Greeks, were thrusting southward into central Greece in 2000BC (Simon 1978, 55). Their dominant passion was fighting, as told by Homer's poetry, which started in the latter half of the eighth century BC.

In the Greek era, the concept of the self started with Homer relating the heroic record of the death of the noble fighters. His great epic shows the turmoil and conflict of human life, reflecting on loneliness, old age and death. The heroes were rewarded by having the history of the deeds they performed recorded and repeated by the poets. The life after death of the Homeric heroes is a world of fleeting shadows drifting endlessly in the underworld. Homer's presentation of the *psuche* (psyche) started with death (Simon 1978, 55). In the *Iliad*, when man is slain, his psyche goes to Hades to continue part of its existence, the corpse being left to be rendered to ashes (Simon 1978, 296; see also Notes 1 and 7 from Chapter 4).

In Book II of the *Odyssey*, Homer provides us with a description of the existence of the psyche in Hades (Simon 1978, 296). The dialogue between Odysseus and the psyche of Achilles in Hades reflects a dreary and joyless existence. It is a flitting shadow on the stage with no power to project itself; it can only speak and be witty after drinking the blood of slain animals. This shows the infinity of being, the release of the psyche after death. It also indicates that the dead heroes were worshipped and that animal sacrifices were performed for them. The psyche in Homer is a sacred thing in that we have faith in it and can swear by it, but it is only a human quality.

Homer does not associate the self with either the physical or the mental (Simon 1978, 60). Emotion, thinking and mental functioning are an amalgam of the mind and the heart. The *phrenes* (mind or wits) signify the diaphragm or the lungs, the *thumos* is an entity or organ that swells within the person, and the *noos* is the agency or the part that sees ahead and plans, also being designated as the plan itself. The *thumos* is also taken to be the locus of impulse and the impulse itself. Homer uses the terms of the warriors to describe the body in the form of organs damaged by fighting, and limbs, muscles, joints and bones as the places of trauma.

The Homeric view portrays the self as being under the control of external forces, the ability to sing, for example, arising because the gods have given the song and lyre. Hard work and winning wars is attribut-able to divine power: in Book XIII of the *Iliad*, Ajax of Oileus and Ajax the son of Telamon drove off the Trojans after they had been possessed by Poseidon, who came down to encourage them to repel the Trojan onslaught (Simon 1978, 64). This outside agency can also take the form of other people, drugs or strong emotion.

The resolve to act thus does not arise from an isolated ego but from the open force field defined by the gods, the group leader being merely a mouthpiece (Zeller 1963, 8). What makes the ego an open force field in Homer's writings is the absence of a structure of or boundaries to the self. We are not private entities; there is no space between individuals. Instead, there exists an interlocking of selves as if we are possessed by and chained to the each other's decisions. Others are our courage, force and action, 'I' standing for the group that has the power to decide, not the individual.

In the Homeric sense, the 'I' self is a collection of the *thumos* (spirit), *kradi* (the heart), *phrenes* or intellect (diaphragm or lungs), *noos* (mental activities) and *menos* or strength (the limbs), courage and an infusion of the gods and our interactive process. To Homer, we are a one in a group, no one being alone. Homer, however, does not portray us as entirely passive, placing us instead in a state of ambivalence when taking decisions. Conflict at a time of action can be seen as a kind of madness in the drama of Homer. After all, it was this content and terminology that Freud used to give force to his views on conflicts and complexes, the Oedipus complex for example.

Homer views life in the sun as the only one truly active against the shadow existence in Hades. In the sunny world, the warrior's mind (*noos*) is superior to his will. Homer calls character 'knowledge', in that a king knows justice, a woman knows chastity, and the hate that filled Achilles knows wrath like a lion. This is the wrath of revenge for his relative, and it is the only cure for his family's grief. The will to act is the force of being possessed by gods. In Homer, the body trained on Olympus is mortal and the soul eternal, the self being portrayed as a social construction of the norms of the community (Zeller 1963, 27; Barnes 1987, 61–70).

After Homer, the Greek philosophy of the self began to take on the form of science based on observation, including astronomy, mathematics, religion and medicine. Nature was seen as animate, the land, sea, mountains, rivers, trees and bushes viewed as forms of the divine beings. Thales (624–546BC), the first to use mathematics to direct his journey, proposed with the hypothesis that water is the main component of living things, but, like Homer, he believed that the determination of being lay in the hands of the gods. Anaximander developed the theory of Thales to include physics in making the body a formation of the opposites warm and cold, which form moisture, and air and fire, these in turn combining to create life.

The Pythagoreans, albeit concerned with body chemistry, maintained their views on the transmigration of the soul. Their aim was to free the body from the circle of birth and to enter into the last divine state of bliss by purification from sensuality and the renunciation of earthly rights. The way to achieve bliss was through rituals, intellectualism and morals.

Part of the process of purification was to abstain from fleshy food and certain types of bean. Life was to be taken extremely seriously, and systematic training was needed for correct conduct. This training involved silence, detachment from others and daily examination. The highest form of purification was considered to be mental work as it was perceived to liberate the soul. Other techniques added for caring for the self were music, gymnastics and vegetarianism as meat disturbed the soul. The Pythagoreans viewed the body as being inferior to the eternal soul. The body was, however, seen as the instrument through which the mind could be accessed. To achieve this aim of purification of the mind, the body was to be hardened by gymnastics, medicine and music (Zeller 1963, 37–8).

The way to purification lay along an ascending road, in that the hardening system for a bard (a commoner) differed from that for a noble philosopher or physician. The noble ones were considered to be nearer the state of bliss in the process of transmigration of the soul, the bard having to progress further to reach the top of the pyramid. In this view of a scale of self-development, we can see that Maslow's pyramid of self-actualization is nearer to the view of the Greeks than was the Vedic approach.

Long before Hippocrates, the Pythagoreans had started rocking the cradle of scientific medicine. Alcmaeon, following the Egyptian path of physiology, was the first Greek to dissect animals and recognize the brain (see Jones 1946) as the central organ of mental life. Philolaus was to postulate that the cause of all illness was to be found in the bodily juices, the blood, the gallbladder and the phlegm. He followed Alcmaeon in the view that illness arose from an imbalance in the powers of opposites, in that one quality was stronger than the other.

Heraclitus (544–484BC) was to dismiss this power of opposites as being unduly negative. He considered that knowledge came from friction and that it is by confronting the opposites in life that we produce knowledge from reason. Heraclitus's approach was to work at both the positive and the negative since he believed that knowledge of the self is formed by feedback from both these aspects. Ethically, he believed in confronting and supporting the law with the same force that we use to defend the nation's sanitary principles.

Empedocles, the Pythagorean who was famous for joining two rivers together in order to create a flood, and later burned out the malaria surrounding the boggy areas of rivers, was to locate the soul in the blood. He saw disease as being of the blood, his prescribed treatment being drugs. Empedocles' advice to medicine was to learn all the drugs that can care for us from the cradle to the grave (Harris 1973, 5–7, 13). To achieve this, medicine must make use of all the sciences and should not confine itself to observation.

Empedocles made the organs the agents of the self (Zeller 1963, 82). The four major organs he identified were:

- the brain, the seat of consciousness, the residence of the mind, which signified the ruling principles;
- the heart, the vital principle of sensation identified with the animals;
- the navel, representing plant qualities;
- the genitals, pertaining to all as we sprout from the sperm.

The Pythagoreans also claimed that the seed carries all the qualities and determines the way in which we are going to develop.

The presentation of the self from the Homeric and post-Homeric time is similar to that of the Vedic version in so far as the soul has an infinite power and the gods are still in control of the will. It has also modelled itself on the Egyptian view in that the mind has been located in the bodily organs. The humoral theory of the Egyptians regarding the source of illness still reigned, with the exception of Homer, who identified emotional conflict. The power of the opposite forces was introduced, the autocracy of one of the opposing forces producing the equation of illness.

It is with Socrates (427–347BC) that the modern view of the self begins to be elaborated. Socrates saw human beings as individuals and as being social, with culture created by language. It is religion, education, art, poetry, ethics, politics and the physical state of the republic that forms the citizens.

Our capacity to change occurs through the acquisition of knowledge. The self is to be developed towards reason through education; to be engaged in public life requires extensive knowledge, and knowledge is only valuable if it is of practical use and is applied ethically. Reason then becomes the foundation of character formation and the basis of citizenship. Like the Pythagoreans, Socrates saw education as a noble process cultivating natural gifts. Learning, if it were to be of any use in character formation, was to begin at a young age and carry on well into the forties for those charged with the responsibility of political life, as education does not sprout unless a depth of knowledge is reached (Plato 1974, 149–50, 392d).

Socrates formed up his plan for citizenship of the republic with knowledge at its head. The plan for the development of the self was to be strongly influenced by and based upon the culture's inherited content. To Socrates, the content of our world is decided by our past, present and future. It is how that content is arranged, the way in which it is formed and presented, that influences our development.

Socrates was conscious of how education can leave a permanent mark on the character (Plato 1974, 147, 391, b,c,d), so his programme is one that is directed at the forms that education should adopt, taking into account the social structure and literature of his time. The content should be purely descriptive, and stories about the gods being evil should be censured. Homer's description of life in Hades, the fight between relatives and the description of rape and sexual abuse between kin should be excluded from literature and the education of young children (Plato 1974, 157, 398b). At an early stage of development, the young should be exposed to guardians who are self-controlled so that children can take from them their cues on how to become perfect citizens. The guardians should be severe rather than amusing, portraying the style of a good person who abides by the principles laid down for him or her (Plato 1974, 150–1, 393b,c,d,e).

In describing the situation to children, the guardians should be aware that the style of presenting the story will influence the audience, and here Socrates rejected the acting form of teaching as he felt that its task was to be descriptive. He wanted guardians to be in a teaching situation where they described the content but did not place themselves as part of the events they were recounting (Plato 1974, 157, 398e). The guardians should show a style of self-detachment and should allow the text to speak for itself. The style of the content and its presentation should be uniform, with an appropriate mode of rhythm to accompany it. Socrates rejected the extreme of the opposites. He wanted the self to be a pandora, a moderator; everything should be taken in moderation.

The content of music was to receive the same treatment as that of literature. The mode and rhythm should suit the words. Lydian music, which is mournful in modes, was to be discouraged (Plato 1974, 162, 401b,c,d,e), and control should be imposed over music and poetry to protect the young citizen.

Mathematics and science were to be left for the latter stage of education by the guardian. Socrates asked for a co-ordination of words, rhythm and mode as it is an awareness of what is goodness that assists in forming the mind and character of the young. He saw that grazing wildly in an unhealthy pasture culminated in psychological damage (Plato 1974, 163, 402b,c).

Youth was seen as an age at which education was crucial. Socrates wanted a clear demarcation to prevent ambiguity so that it should be presented in an unequivocal manner; only the value of beauty was to be presented. By learning what is good and beautiful at an early age, we will have cognisance of how to differentiate these from that which is bad (Plato 1974, 163, 402b,c).

The message that Socrates was conveying is that the content, style and representation of what we expose children to at an early stage of development will influence them later on in life. Exposing youth to violence, ugliness and rape scenes is what will form the drama of the child, culminating in conflict. It is this permanent mark of pain left on the character which Freud addressed himself to, this primal scene of painful learning resulting in psychological trauma.

Socrates' approach is to point out clearly which form and direction education should take. He considered a liberal education as being the form that drives the medical profession to a medical nemesis to identify conditions since, for Socrates, madness can be a failure of social cognition (Plato 1974, 166, 403d). The new names for diseases themselves force the judges to come and deal with deviants.

The form of knowledge prescribed is what goes to produce the best physique. The supremacy of education and knowledge that goes to form a refinely trained mind is the controller of physique, so that once the character is formed, physical training needs only a rough outline (Plato 1974, 166, 403e). The guardian involved in training should be forbidden to drink as it affects the memory.

Diet and sleep are seen as being the most important factors in creating a healthy and delicate balance, deviation from either of these two possibly leading to serious illness (Plato 1974, 167, 404e). For physical fitness for the general public, Socrates advocated a miniature style of military training.

As for luxuries such as Corinthian girlfriends and Attic confectionery, these meant to be enjoyed in harmonious rhythm with the principle of moderation, as also applied to poetry and music (Plato 1974, 168, 405). Socrates believed that a lack of regard to food produced disease, the opening of surgeries, as well as indiscipline in character, keeping the lawyers busy. Within the republic, the doctors were in charge of the body in case of illness, the lawyers dealt with the law-breakers, and the philosophers became the rulers responsible for the process of education. Socrates portrayed the gods as being all that involves goodness, and replaced the power of control in the republic by that of human beings.

The plan for education having been drawn up, Socrates had to decide whom to educate. Following his vision that we are derived from the elements of the soil, he employed a metallurgical form of classification (Plato 1974, 182, 415c), arranging society in a hierarchical fashion in the order of:

- the Gold, qualified from birth to be rulers;
- the Silver, the auxiliaries, whose task it is to assist the rulers in planning and decision-making.
- the Iron and the Bronze, the farmers and manual workers, the 'muscle'.

The individual is born with one of these qualities, the natural part, but education and the social situation are what will distil, refine and make the Gold and Silver ones shine. It is the responsibility of the family to watch and observe their offspring and to detect whether one of their children is born with such qualities. This will display itself in how the child deals and copes successfully with stressful situations. Parents with one quality may produce children of different metallic properties, the advice Socrates gave to them being that they should be prepared to let the child move to his or her appropriate level (Zeller 1963, 45).

Once the selection has been made, the process of self-purification takes on the Socratic gaze, which is the application of the principle of moderation and the avoidance of the dramatic Homeric approach. Scenes or styles of violence are not allowed until a certain level of consciousness is reached, allowing the person to differentiate between goodness and badness. It is how the three groups are educated, each according to its natural potential, which gives us the Socratic form of the soul or the self.

Socrates defined each one of us as representing in ourselves the constitution of the republic, and he was much concerned with refining the role of the guardians. His main interest lay with the process and the style of how things are displayed and what the constant, natural qualities should be. Producing disciplined and controlled guardians would lead to the republic Socrates wanted; they could be seen as the future planners, the mentors who assist us in tracing our path in the jungle of life.

The checklist for the guardians involved certain qualities as well as their form of education. The guardians had to have great skills besides intelligence and needed to be caring towards the community. Their training involved taking on the hardest and most courageous tasks. The test of endurance involved having the skill, knowledge and strength of determination to dive to the bottom of the sea, enter a dark cave where no light ever shone, a blind world, and surface with a blind eel, suffering no discomfort to themselves or their blind captive. This noble one had to be a 'Delian diver', someone with faith in his experience and skills (Plato 1974, 180, 413 c,d).

This demanded great technique and depth of knowledge, as well as the ability to maintain a balance of harmony with the self and others. Socrates saw his guardians as existing in relation to others, there being no place for egoism. The guardians were to obey the principles of what was best for the constitution, and any sign of deviation from this commitment when under stress was a weakness that was watched for during their education (Plato 1974, 278, 486).

To ensure the development of these qualities, Socrates placed his guardians in a place free from temptation so that they could lead a communal life with no material property (Plato 1974, 183, 416b). They were to be provided for and properly educated in order to prevent their becoming 'wild ravenous dogs' (Plato 1974, 183, 416b). Their education, meditation and principles were what was to lead to wisdom and foresight. This was the form that would provide harmony between the three sections of the republic, as a state of disharmony would lead to constitutional chaos.

Socrates believed in keeping the three groups separate from each other, as crossing and mingling in each other's affairs would lead to conflict. He commented that, 'The discipline must influence private and public life to such a degree that the child will identify things when they go wrong', and 'A good citizen does not have to worry about the Law, he is embodied in it' (Plato 1974, 193, 425).

The rulers were to be selected to form a minority group. With Socrates, the guardians' skills, experiences and state of harmony placed them above the others; they were the super-ego ruling the other two forces. The way in which this super-ego displayed itself was held to be by honesty and openness (Plato 1974, 412e, 413). With Socrates's open book approach, the difference between the private and public self is that of transcendence. The public self is transcendent in so far as it is in the world through commitment, faith and respect, an ethical approach being the necessary consequence of reflection. Reflection is being in the world, the republic, and it is indicated through skilful action according to the prescribed educational principles.

Socrates made us controllers of our own destiny under the possession or gaze of education and experience, along with the supporting qualities of respect, commitment, understanding and principles of care, the emotional toning that produces harmony of the self. In the process of attunement and harmony, we also become aware of others. We are inevitably with other people, but there will always be a 'gap' between each of us in that we are at different levels of consciousness. Socrates made us aware of the problems that may develop if any one of the group is left in charge or if insufficient consultation takes place. Mediation means listening to all sides of the argument before establishing moderation and harmony.

When we are involved in action or decision-making in which there is no conflict of interest, our action is a voluntary one (Plato 1974, 209, 435e). The problem arises when carrying out the act involves some conflict that influences the economy of the self, thus meaning that one of the parties has to surrender the asset to the other side. In a case where the economy of self is likely to suffer, the act becomes involuntary in that we have to bring our principles, knowledge, skills and experiences to the task, thus clearing our doubts before acting.

This skill of self-harmony involves the use of our senses and experiences and having faith in what we have learned and experienced as a basis for self-assertion. This power of assertion is the self gathering its forces, which involves respect, self-discipline and bravery, the reasoning of power of the self. Plato stated, 'the spirit is what holds fast to order and reason, about what things ought to be in spite of pain and this is the smart part as it decides what is best for the three' (Plato 1974, 220, 442 c,d).

Socrates stated that this is the third element of the self, the ego having the function of mastery. This third element of the self is characterized as a warrior, as reasoning is a state of war within the self. We have to pass through a state of self-disturbance before establishing tranquillity. In some cases, when we know that we are right to act in a certain way and are prevented from doing so, the third element will boil with indignation, and there will come into force to exert the will those qualities whose task it is to assist in the decision-making.

But the fight to victory is not one of a free will that can do as it pleases. Reasoning, in the Socratic form, involves discipline, principle and education with qualities of goodness, operating in response to the demands of particular situations. It is like a judge who has to bring into operation the training skills, knowledge and principles of what is goodness and badness before he can act (Plato 1974, 216, 446d). This third element is the force that can mediate and legislate to bring harmony between the other two groups. The defeat of this element thus brings open and unresolved conflict, which will affect both the constitution and the republic.

The third element is not isolated from the other two as it may decide to carry out a desire that is not acceptable (there being no place for egotism in Socrates's republic). So the third element is involved in the first element and part of the lowest element. Socrates makes it clear that the third element is trained alongside the guardian (the super-ego) and that the third element and the lowest element, Iron and Bronze, should never be left in charge. The warrior organizes the lowest layers so must have some insight into their needs.

In Book VIII of *The Republic*, Socrates makes us aware of the imperfect society and the havoc it may cause. Freud, too, saw the self as tripartite and as expressing conflict within society. The Socratic and Freudian views are, however, not identical, for the super-ego (guardian) under the Socratic gaze can be seen as the universal consciousness that is formed from ethical deliberations, and the third element, the ego, is the individual using the lower unconscious substance, experience and the principle of caring of the guardian to deal with the reality of our social situations.

The environment

Greek philosophers prior to the late Pythagoreans considered the whole environment, including human beings, to be possessed by the gods. Pythagoreans saw the forest as the place for non-attachment, seclusion and meditation. It was in fact so important that Aristotle, in his classification of science renamed the environment as that of Egypt accorded to the body shape the powerful odd mathematical number seven (Jones 1946, 7).

We have already seen how this conception of the environment changed in favour of a scientific one, particularly following Empedocles, who saw life as a balance between *milieu* and organisms (Barker 1929). He ordered doctors to become involved in regional surveys, the climate, water supply, vegetation and geographical areas where people lived coming under the medical gaze. As geography and environment influence the body, certain diseases are to be found in certain climatic conditions. We have to control our environment by the power of scientific knowledge. In *Littre* Volume 2 (Barker 1929), medicine was to take account of the meteorology of the wind and the quality and texture of water when dealing with disease. The approach of the scientific therapeutic gaze thus commenced.

Ethical perspective

Although we clearly see the beginning of the scientific approach to illness in Greek times, this view co-existed alongside the earlier views of illness as being possession by gods. Both science and demonic possession can in a sense be regarded as deterministic models, and it is only with Socrates that questions of the self as a rational and moral being entered into the equation.

The co-existence of science and the gods can be seen in the early Greek perspective, as described above. As we have seen, Homer described the psyche as starting with death. The joylessness of death could be rendered powerful and full of intelligence after consuming the blood of slain animals through a system of worshipping.

Homer left the power of the self in the hands of the divine and saw the ego as an open force field, the agency of action being the power of the gods. He saw character as knowledge and power as action in that a king knows justice, a woman knows chastity and the hate-filled Achilles knows the wrath of revenge, like a lion. Homer placed us in an ethical triangle of determinism: on the one side our power to act, fight and sing is defined by the gods; on the other, the power of the self depends on our action in that only the warriors were praised for their deeds, and their power depended on resolving conflict. There is no censorship in Homer; he exposes the violence of the bedroom scene and the fights amongst the gods and leaves it to us to resolve and confront the situation.

Homer saw ethics as action involving not only conscious action during our lifetime, but also the deeds as narrated in Hades. He saw the ashes of the dead warriors influencing the actions of the poets. Actions go beyond the power of the lens and the blindness of the retina into the dark path of our embodiment, involving our historicity before and after death. Transcendence is the deconstruction of our deeds, of which we may or may not be conscious.

Homer did not, however, leave our actions completely in the hands of the gods as he made us aware of the conflict of interest, which could lead to madness in cases of ambivalence. The agent, in the Homerian view, could be seen as an amalgam consisting of the spirit of consciousness, our past experience in a previous life, and character or intellect, which is an infusion of godliness and the power to resolve conflict. The self as an agent is in a sense an amalgam of these three perspectives.

Pythagoras, who is often seen as the founder of the Hippocratic Oath, envisaged the freeing of the self through a process of purification of the body by diet, systematic training and silence (Edelstein 1967, 9–57). This involved being away from others in the forest for daily introspection, which was to lead to the liberation of the soul. The Pythagorean ethic was not only concerned with consciousness training, but also consisted of correct behaviour, diet and environment. The philosopher-physician was to be concerned with the body, the soul and the environment. Self-purification occurred on a developmental level in that Pythagoreans used a scaling system, the philosopher-physician having achieved the highest level of consciousness (Edelstein 1967, 37).

People were to be dealt with according to their level of refinement as a commoner could not be dealt with in the same way as a philosopher or a physician. Ethical and self-purification leads to knowledge and a higher level of consciousness. The style of self-purification proposed involved silence, silence not only in being alone with oneself but also in proper communication with others.

In relationships with other people, the Pythagoreans argued that it was possible to take a well-timed or an ill-timed attitude. Speech and actions were to vary according to the circumstances and the situation of those concerned. This would result in timeliness, appropriateness and fitness of behaviour, which would in turn reveal good manners. The philosopher-physician was to take account of the patient's daily activity and keep to himself all that was seen and heard. The Pythagorean school sets the rules regarding communication, in that silence, a respectful attitude, confidentiality and taking into account what the patient did in the daily event became the ground rules of communication.

The revolutionary shift from the view of self as being possessed by the gods had already started. The ethical base moved from being controlled by the gods to being controlled by the environment. The body, in the Egyptian and Pythagorean times, became an interactive one. The Egyptians and Pythagoreans laid down the ground rules under which therapeutic intervention should take place (Edelstein 1967, 37).

Socrates saw education as valuable when applied ethically. He was concerned with the process that education should take in the formation of the citizen. Since children should not be exposed to painful drama, Homer's description of violence and painful experiences and the account of violence between the gods were to be excluded. The guardians or teachers to whom children were to be exposed needed to be perfect citizens as they were responsible for providing cues for such perfect citizenship.

Education involving music, literature, physical training and diet was to follow the principle of coordination and rhythm. Grazing in an 'unhealthy wild pasture' culminated in psychological damage and was seen as the origin of indiscipline and disease. Under Socrates, education and knowledge thus became the way forward to human development, with an emphasis on respect, self-discipline and courage. This became the source that activated reflective, mediative thinking and autonomous power. Socrates placed ethics on a societal level in that he was concerned with a situation and with the process of taking care over what was presented, especially to children.

Views of madness

The self, as described above, was in the Greek perspective viewed as the physical body threaded through by the elements of the environment. The bodily mesh was formed from what was ingested from the surroundings. The power of the self and the intellect was an aspect of the body fluid, the blood circulating through the heart muscles. The source of madness itself was seen as being the vagrant element of the blood.

Divine power still affected the individual in that the power to win wars and to sing, for example, was believed to be under the influence of the gods. Homer presented the self as developing from conflicting situations, and to Socrates education was the form of the self. The five poles – the body, the environment, the situational factors, education and the gods, which formed the bonding of the self – were also responsible for sources of illness. The Greeks' view of madness took into account these five poles, which cannot be seen in isolation from each other but are instead cemented together in that the self was seen as the organism and the environment.

The Greek perspective on madness was an elaboration of Egyptian, Oriental and Asian views (Whittaker 1961). These authors pointed out that there was a kind of universality in archaic medicine in that the practices of most countries were similar. According to these writers, the Egyptian and Mesopotamian approaches to medicine were fused together with the Greek approach and translated into Greek and Latin under the approach of Hippocrates. This led to the institution of medicine for five centuries before Christ and nearly a dozen afterwards.

What were considered to be the sources of madness during that time have already been described. Like the other approaches, that of the Greeks left us in the power of god, the environment, minerals, water and natural elements. Education became a powerful source of self-power, but the gods was held responsible for long-term life situations. The essential elements of existence were, however, still to be found in the earthly environment.

Alcamaeon of Croton, the first person to dissect the brain, identified it as the central organ of the sensory system. He commented that when imbalances were created in the system of opposing elements, disease resulted. This became known as the doctrine of the Golden Mean. Alcamaeon and Anaxinenes developed the doctrine that the human being was a sort of miniature world and that this human microcosm lay in a direct relationship, in terms of composition and functioning, with the macrocosm, which is the universe itself. This reflects the universality of being.

The biochemical view of Alcamaeon described earlier was further developed by Empedocles, who formulated that the four elements – fire, air, water and earth – were the authorities of health. Empedocles' thesis was that we should be able to identify the source of madness or illness by examining a single unit, a cell of the human body, and that drugs would be the agent of medical management. The practice of medicine and administration of drugs were to be controlled by code of law, and the four humours were still held to be responsible for illness and madness.

The biological sources or pathological aspects of disease having been identified at an organic and environmental level, the next development was to view society itself as being partly responsible for the manufacture of disorders. Socrates' views were that society should be educated and everything should occur in moderation and be controlled. An exposure to violence led to violence, so children should not be exposed to stories of sexual acts and violence amongst the gods. The media, including children's literature, had to be censored. Music, exercises and outdoor activities became the order of the day for a healthy individual and society; laxity in these disciplines was what kept the doctors and the court busy.

Education was to be approached seriously, taking into account the qualities and ability of the pupils. The assessment of human dimensions thus started and still affects the schooling system and the assessment for mental health management. Socrates was, however, not only interested in assessment and the end-product, his main concern being the process through which the individual had to go. Here he placed the responsibility into the hands of the mentors and the individual. Process was not only what the mentor did, but also how the individual arranged what was given. In this way, Socrates held the individual responsible for his or her own development.

Faith had thus moved from the gods to human qualities. Human beings were now in control, although the gods still inhabited them, especially in the case of chronic illness. The self became an amalgam of god, social training, self-discipline, biology and the environment. A disturbance in any of these forces would result in social disorders or diseases. Conflict in society and the individual resulting from excess became a kind of madness. The foundations for the approaches to psychology and psychiatry had in this way been laid; the management of how to prevent disease and social disorders in the form of education and self control was on its way.

The first mental hospital or lunatic asylum was built in Baghdad between the sixth and the ninth centuries AD, and the first attendants appointed. There is very little direct information on how the mad were treated, but we do know that there was no distinction made between the treatment of physical and mental illness. In both cases, bleeding and cleansing of the body were the major forms of treatment. There is no evidence of institutionalized control except for Greek times when 'vagabonds' and 'deviants' were imprisoned alongside criminals.

Continuities and contradiction in ancient 'psychiatry'

Not surprisingly perhaps, the evidence for similarities between the three cultures we have discussed is very strong, and this will be reviewed below. At the same time, I shall argue that there emerges over time the foundation of a modern contradiction in the view of madness and its management. On the one hand, the development of medicine and a deterministic view of the human body was associated with purely mechanical forms of treatment, such as blood-letting and cleansing of the body. On the other hand, there is a strong emphasis in Vedantic and later Greek perspectives on social and individual responsibility for human well-being.

It can of course be argued that, at one level, our capacity to see ourselves as determinate objects is part of the very process of taking responsibility for ourselves through acts of reason. In terms of the ways in which madness is regarded, however, it is reasonable to talk of a contradiction, an unresolved tension, that persists to the present day and has made caring for madness an often ambivalent process. This is, in short, the question of whether we are to regard the patient as an object to be treated using various physical interventions or as a person who needs to take responsibility for his or her development. How this question is answered helps to determine the kind of philosophy of caring that informs the training of the psychiatric nurse. It is to this issue that I shall turn in Section III of this text.

Let us start by examining the similarities we have observed. The crisis of continuities and contradiction will adopt the following form:

- Continuities
- An abiding problem.

Continuities

One of the major similarities displayed by the three cultures is an emphasis on nature as consisting of opposing forces that need to be held in balance for a healthy life. The Vedic culture presented the view of the self as being positive and negative, these opposing forces also being associated with the power of the self and language, Krishna, being the positive force, and Shiva the negative pole or the destroyer. The force of language was viewed as being a form of friction between these two forces.

The Egyptians saw the Nile as the instigator of biological conflict and the source of tension in that the Nile's water was both the life blood and the poison of Egypt. It could make the nation flourish, but it could also lead to madness and death through malaria and other diseases associated with the black, the green and the red bile (the blood humours). The social environment of the Nile created tension in how women of different social classes were treated.

This loving and rocky relationship with the Nile produced a form of sociology based on social class, gender and economy. The Nile represented the beauty of the woman, who, for Aristotle, possessed the most powerful odd number, the number seven; it was life and death, disease, wealth, sexuality and politics. It was the Egyptian passion with the Nile that made her the symbolic mother, the womb of Egypt, whose blood could feed the nation through her network of capillaries and canaliculi, but who could, when in a rage, destroy the population. She was thus the ambivalence of the caring/destroying mother. The Egyptians went further, humanizing and personifying Egypt, the Red and Black seas forming the legs, the Nile being the uterus and the land of Egypt the body. They saw humans as being essentially a part of their surroundings, a view they shared with the Greeks and Vedics. What love and treatment the surroundings received were to be passed on to the children of the Nile, as woman, in the form of the curing or prevention of illness, including surgery, drilling, burning, fumigating and anasthemosis to control the rage, and shaving to prevent germs breeding.

This view of opposites also took the form of a physics postulating forms of friction such as cold/hot and creativity/destruction, which were the climatic elements that gave madness and the self a form. From this physics, the Egyptians moved to similarities in chemistry. They believed that humans consisted of the blood enzymes and the humours, which originated from the bile of the soil or water supply. These chemicals, when in the blood, could cause madness and disease. The Egyptians and the Greeks gave us a biological form in that the organs were measured and the body was said to be guarded by god. The Vedic perceived that the most powerful gods guarded the brain and the sexual organs.

The idea of opposites took on mathematical expression: the self was not only seen in the form of opposites, but also became a kind of pairing of opposites, the opposite odd numbers being more powerful. This mathematical form of opposites influenced the three cultures. Heraclitus advocated that reason, upon which knowledge is based, originated from the friction of the opposites. Empirical science used observation and mathematics to give form to man's observations in the Egyptian and Greeks cultures, Thale arguing that we are 90% water and need air and water to create movement.

These ancient cultures had a passion to form an understanding of their environment. The rivers and forests were held to be places of meditation. It was through caring for the environment, eliminating toxic material and not poisoning the water and food supply that we would produce healthy physical beings. (This point was also made by

Tuke in 1803 in addressing the caring of madness, his view being that we should save the 'bark of being' from the cruel environment of the private madhouse, thus acknowledging the value of a caring and therapeutic environment.) We were already warned by the Vedic and the Greek cultures that meat in excess and certain vegetables caused madness.

Science gradually supplanted the power of the gods, leading to a perception of the body as chemical and physical elements, frictions and biochemical abnormalities. A class system, a psychosexual politics and form of environmental control, and the birth of the disembodiment of experience by the ancient sciences had started. The delivery of this baby took a long time, not occurring until the time of the Enlightenment. The mathematical expression of pairing opposing forces and measurement was also to influence our perception. A consensus emerges here on the nature of madness, an agreement that there was a strong link between humour in the blood, which originated from the environment and food supply, and illness.

An abiding problem

We have, however, also seen how, with the decline of divine intervention, there occurred a shift towards social and individual responsibility, especially in Socratic teachings with its influence of ethics and education. The Greek world wanted responsible citizens, demanding respect and commitment in action and interaction. Freedom carried with it responsibility and care for oneself and others so there was no place for egotism.

The Vedic and Greek cultures had a similar ethics of the self. They saw training and education, along with commitment and responsibility, as being the foundation of autonomy and the development of the self. They were concerned with developing, redirecting and strengthening their citizens or community members. Unattachment, meditation and educational process, as shown by the mentors and guardians, were the means of forming the citizen. Socrates prescribed training and emotional and social control through censorship and mediation. Everything was to occur in moderation in order to maintain control, prevent criminal action and stop the child becoming delinquent through exposure to criminal acts. The lack of self-control could be seen as madness or social deviance. Like biological blockage, emotional blockage or excess could be seen as the cause of madness. Education and training thus provided the necessary corrective rules for the republic. Socrates, however, respected the individual in that everyone was educated according to his or her ability.

We see, therefore, an increasing concern with human understanding through training and education. An ethical demand laying responsibility on the citizen was established in these three cultures, comprising the conditions for personal development. These conditions now form part of the rules of counselling and psychotherapy. It is thus possible to discern in ancient societies the foundation of the division between natural-scientific and social-ethical approaches to human being and, consequently, also to madness.

The emphasis upon socialization can of course be seen as part of a social-deterministic framework, which is a natural ally to the determinism of the natural sciences. But to assert this view as a complete and sufficient explanation of human behaviour is to ignore the Socratic message that it is individuals who need to take responsibility for themselves through understanding, which will in turn propel them to right action. This, as we well know today, leads to a quite different approach to madness – one based upon insight and personal development rather than drugs.

These conflicts are of critical importance for the role of the psychiatric nurse, who may find him- or herself asked to be both an attendant in the administration of a medical model and a carer for the patient's personal development. This theme will be revisited in Section III.

Chapter 4

From the Enlightenment to the present

An account of care

From the time of ancient history through the Dark Ages and the Renaissance, very few changes took place in the treatment of madness, as Porter (1985) has pointed out. The principles and ideology of management are similar to the Greek model even today as intervention is still related to the blood and its impurities, together with cognitive and social control. Development has taken the form of a refinement of the techniques to harness or eliminate madness. Whereas in the past the mad were free to roam or remain with their family and community, the period under review saw them increasingly placed in institutions. Foucault (1961, 46–64) pointed out that the mad, the criminal and those with other illnesses were like a ship without the mast, and they were placed in similar institutions. These houses were, according to Foucault, no more than prisons for social nuisances.

The history of the management of madness by fumigating, bleeding at certain seasons of the year, blistering, leeching and surgical application carried on during institutionalization. The other form of management that became popular was hydrotherapy (Hunter & McAlpine 1963, 254–7), which took the form of hosing, internal lavage and being placed underwater. The measured force of weight and pressure had the aim of forcing the madness out of the sufferer. It was recommended that the mad should be kept under a water pressure of some 20 feet height for 15 minutes. For women, the pressure was 15 tons of water for 30 minutes. In the case of a woman who had left her husband, the treatment could be increased from 30 to 90 minutes, to be administered fully naked until she became an obedient dutiful wife. The other form of water therapy was ducking to identify madness or being possessed.

The seventeenth and eighteenth centuries, the so-called time of Enlightenment, were to change the perception of madness. The revolution in France freed the citizen but not the madman. He or she was still the possession of the sovereign power, whether king or state. In sixteenth-century England, the madmen or poor were thrown out of the monasteries with the breach from Rome in 1532. This created a crisis for Elizabeth I, who had to pass the Vagabond Laws under which those who were homeless were branded on the forehead with a letter V. We also saw the first Community Act of 1601–02, which charged any able bodied person in full employment one penny for management of the poor and sick in their county. At the same time, madness was seen as leading to diminished responsibility, as in the case of William Hackett, who wanted to assassinate the Queen for being a witch and 'white bastard' but was given protection on the grounds of madness (Hunter & McAlpine 1963, 44-5). Madness remained the property of the Crown state in both countries, even though the King was beheaded in France.

The history of the Enlightenment shows the beginning of incarceration of the mad in private clinics and homes in England, although the first mental hospital in London was established at St Mary of Bethlehem, in about 1200. Incarceration can, according to historians, be dated as far back as the ninth or even sixth century AD (Alexander & Selesick 1967, 21; Pillau 1979, 89–90). The first asylum was built near Alexandria, with the appointment of the first attendants.

During the Enlightenment, with the advancement of science, madness moved increasingly under the scientific gaze. Medicine saw significant advances that could be applied to the treatment of the insane. The laws of astronomy were to be applied to determine when bleeding should take place (MacDonald 1981, xii–xiv). The law of pressure and volume could also be applied. Madness was seen as not only being possessed by an enzyme or humour in the blood, but also arising, according to Harvey, from a blockage (Alexander & Selesick 1967, 107). Chemicals such as mercury, iron, zinc and others discovered by that time were to be administered for madness, together with emetics and purgatives (Kraepelin 1962, 60–1).

With the incarceration of madness came exploitation. As Parry-Jones (1972) has pointed out, some were placed into indefinite care so that the proprietors and relatives of the sick could make a fortune. With institutionalization came too the caging and chaining system of care. MacDonald (1981), Porter and Shepherd (1985) and Foucault (1961) have presented us with accounts of the management of madness from the Enlightenment to today (Foucault 1961, Ch 7). Foucault pointed out that the scientific gaze, by which he means biology, physics, chemistry and social sciences as employed by medicine, gives us a disembodied account of madness. Madness was placed under the gaze of these sciences and under what Foucault terms the Panoptican gaze.

It was incarceration and this cruel way of managing madness that made Pinell open a psychiatric hospital for the management of madness in 1814 as reported in Kraepelin (1962, 11). In this system of care, the patient who was cured became the attendant. This approach was to be followed by Tuke in England in 1803, his aim being to support and cure the mad. The routine was cleansing, feeding and spiritual training. The Retreat built by Tuke was to become a model of care. Attendants and matrons were to be selected from those who had been cured (Parry-Jones 1972, 120). Those who possessed the metallic qualities, as advocated by Socrates, were to be selected to become the attendants, the superintendents and the matrons. To improve the standard of the attendants, visitors were invited on a Sunday afternoon to act as social model for them. The hope was that the social graces would then rub off onto the patients during interaction with the attendants.

Such experiments were, however, in the minority as the major emphasis lay on restraint. Restraints and shocks included the use of straightjackets, the spinning chair and the sudden drop. In all cases, argued Jones (1972), the aim was to shock the madness out of the patient. One of the most controversial, electric shock treatment (the electric shock being produced by steam), was used by Wesley as early as 1810.

Management by restraint and chemical control, supported by the legal system, was still dominant in the twentieth century. In 1925, the large institutions were becoming unpopular, and a movement towards the villa system began, the first such establishment to be built being Runwell Hospital. Local authorities and general hospitals were made responsible for the mentally ill. The 1950s saw the introduction of tranquillizers, the powerful chemicals that were to replace the attendant's muscles (Hunter & MacAlpine 1963, 98–9). Social and occupational training started on the shop floor of the asylum in order to provide industrial work to occupy the patients and attendants.

With the passage of further acts and the increasing unpopularity of the asylum, as reflected in the work of Goffman (1961) and Barton (1959), the direction of development pointed towards the community. The 1970s and 80s saw the closure of the large asylums and the move to community care. The insane were to be released once more, but this time properly assessed and well directed (Community Care Act 1990). Currently, however, there are calls for the protection of the community and for mini security systems to hold the insane. Just as the large monasteries and workhouses were to be replaced by private clinics, the big asylums, which once took over from the private clinics, have increasingly been replaced by private clinics, National Health Trust secured units and community care. The asylum has, possibly, become a dinosaur, but it is not clear whether society can do without secure accommodation entirely for those judged dangerous to it.

The role of the attendant has consequently moved from caring in the asylum to that of nursing in the small institution and the community, with a range of therapeutic tools to treat madness. We shall now examine the history of the attendant.

A history of the attendant

Before the institutionalization of madness became widespread, it was clearly the task of the family and community to care as best they could for the insane. Monasteries and convents played their part in caring for the mad alongside the sick, destitute and infirm (Barns 1976; Plomer 1977; Weiner 1993). There were often conflicts between religious carers and medical officers concerning the nature of treatment (Jones 1989). It is interesting to read in Kilvert's diary, written between 1870 and 1879, that many families were, even at this time, looking after mentally ill relatives.

It was the beginning of the asylum that brought the attendant into being. At first, asylums were privately owned. Parry-Jones (1972) points out how an attendant who wrote a diary describing the cruelty in one private house had to flee to America when the diary's content became public (Parry-Jones 1972, 235).

It is clear from the account given by Hunter & McAlpine (1963) of 300 years of psychiatry, that the attendants were responsible for administering treatment when they felt that there was a need for further bleeding. A more positive approach towards the job of the attendant did not come about until the time of Pinell and Tuke in 1814. They advocated the use of ex-patients, who had been cured, as carers; the experience of madness and recovery from the condition were perceived to comprise a powerful force. These ex-patients who became attendants spent day and night on the ward. This residence on the ward meant that they were responsible for 24-hour care whether they were on or off duty.

By and large, however, the attendants were ruled by a strict regime. They were allowed out during weekends, the weekend pass being granted on the discretion of the matron (Carpenter 1980, 123–46). Payment was a few pence a week; free time was limited since it was believed that too much money and spare time would turn the attendant into a lazy and bad-mannered drunk (Adams 1969, 11–26; Carpenter 1980, 131–2).

This oppression became obvious in 1956 when psychiatric nurses asked for a pay rise. The superintendent and parliamentary representative stated that too much money and free time would spoil the attendant, which would affect patient care. Their job was seen as being not too demanding, so they should not be overpaid for enjoying themselves. The attendants were under the control of the owners and superintendent. They had to seek permission even to get married.

The attendants' training consisted of learning from others and from the 'visitors' described above. They were responsible for the daily routine of maintaining control and cleanliness. They assisted in the management of care, the wards and the hospital. As they were also responsible for the industrial work and farming, they were sometimes referred to as 'farmer's labourer' (Cotgrove 1967). They were called upon to control and handle violent patients so recruitment was based on a good body build and, curiously, an interest in music.

Under the direction of the reformist Connelly, in the second part of the 1850s, the attendant took on a more active role (Walker 1954, 101–2). Connelly was one of the first to take an interest in the training of attendants, giving lectures and relating theory to practice. His aim was to establish a skilled nursing force. Connelly fought against mismanagement and cruelty to patients, following the approach of Tukes and Pinel.

The role of restraint and physical control started to diminish with the introduction of training for attendants. The first body responsible for such training was the Association of Psychological Medicine, established at the beginning of the twentieth century, the qualification being an RMPA (Registered Member of the Psychological Association). The first meeting of the Association was held in 1841. The text that was followed was the Red Hand Book (Newington et al 1909), the text dealing mostly with the physical aspect of mental illness, outlining the duties of the attendant in this respect (Newington et al. 1909, 361–72.

The attendants' role, as laid down by this handbook, was to secure the comfort, welfare and safety of patients. Attendants were to be cheerful, gentle, forbearing, patient and humane in speech and action, and to set an example of cleanliness, obedience and industriousness. No deception was to be employed. Violence on the part of patient should never be met with the same conduct. The 1890 Lunacy Act, section 322, made it an offence for the manager or attendant to ill-treat or neglect the patient. Abuse of the patient and ill-treatment was also covered in section 342. Gossip was to be avoided, and a confidentiality clause was introduced. The attendant was also responsible for the asylum environment. The general duties of the attendant covered the whole space of the asylum as well as the external environment surrounding the hospital. The clinic was seen as a therapeutic milieu with the attendant playing a constructive part.

Attendants came under the registration of the General Nursing Council in 1919, and from then on the Council was responsible for the training of psychiatric nurses. The Horder (RCN, 1942) and Wood (1947) Reports, which looked at nursing in 1942, recognized the need for training and recommended an 18-month training involving 6 months of specialist skills (Ramprogus 1995, 4). This view was rejected by the matrons, who preferred the 3-year training. From that time until late 1980s, the training of nurses lay in the hands of the matron and health authorities. With the introduction of Project 2000, such training became the responsibility of higher education and the United Kingdom Central Council for Nursing, Midwifery and Health Visiting (UKCC). This body is responsible for registering, maintaining a register and controlling and monitoring members' progress for the benefit of the public.

With the change in the management of care in recent times, mental health nurses have yet again changed their role. The introduction of tranquillizers and the closure of the asylum did not lead to the death of the attendant. Instead, mental health nurses now became members of the mental health multidisciplinary team, taking part in chemotherapy, cognitive control and social training. They are thus representatives of the health authority responsible for implementing the policies and the Mental Health Act in the interests of the patient. As described above, the attendant/mental health nurse operated throughout the clinic in a multidisciplinary therapeutic milieu. This has, perhaps, led to a more fragmented approach, which needs much attention to achieve coherence in practice.

Summary

In this section, I have reviewed the history of our understanding of madness and of caring for madness. I have placed particular emphasis on the ancient history of the Vedic, Egyptian and Greek civilizations since these have very largely defined the parameters within which we still work today. In particular, the growth of a mechanical, scientific approach to madness has been the dominant influence, although it must be said that most mechanical interventions have had little basis in reliable science. At the same time, the importance of personal development and self-control sits somewhat uneasily alongside the traditional medical model (witness the counter-articles from such authors as Rogers 1965, Szasz 1961 and Laing 1960). The role of the psychiatric nurse thus encompasses both physical treatment and psychological development. This thesis is concerned with the latter and particularly with how nurses learn from their experiences in terms of both their own development and their exposure to patients.

The history of psychiatry does not have a great deal to say about the role of the attendant. This section has shown this role is a complex one, and in the next section I examine how students in training learn to cope with it. Present practice and attitudes are, however, clearly rooted in the past, and we would therefore expect to see certain continuities between the historical account of Section I and students' experiences as reported in Section II. The role of the psychiatric nurse remains very much defined in the context of the medical model. I am not, however, arguing for any strictly deterministic view, since it is probable that each generation of students must learn to find its own way of meeting the task of caring for madness.

'I believe that my originality, (if that is the right word), is an originality belonging to the soil rather than the seed. (Perhaps I have no seed of my own). Sow a seed in my soil and it will grow differently than it would in any other soil'.

Wittgenstein, L., (1939-40, p.25 from McGuiness, B., 1982).

Section II

Experiencing Training – Students' Accounts of the Process of Becoming a Registered Mental Nurse

Chapter 5
Study background

There is something I don't know
that I am supposed to know.
I don't know what it is I don't know
and yet I'm supposed to know
and I feel I look stupid
if I seem both not to know it
and not know what it is I don't know.

This is nerve-racking
since I don't know what I must pretend to know.
Therefore I pretend to know everything.

I feel you know what I am supposed to know
but you can't tell me what it is
because you don't know that I don't know what it is.

You may know what I don't know but not that I
don't know it,
and I can't tell you so you will have to tell me
everything.

(Laing 1976)

Three students (BAC, LO and LA) quoted the passage from R.D. Laing's work in order to express their feelings about their course of training, saying that 'this poem seems to sum up how we felt about our first year, especially experiential learning'. Such perplexity is not uncommon.

Section I presented an historical account of how madness has been managed throughout the ages and of the developing role of what we now call the mental health nurse. In this section, students' accounts of their experiences during training will be based very largely upon the categories deriving from this historical account.

We saw that the process of becoming a lunatic attendant was a development from the first-hand experience of madness to being cured from the condition with care. Experiencing madness, confronting it and reflecting upon it under supervision of the lunatic attendants (previously mad themselves), and then making use of that experience to project it in a caring situation, defined the role of attending. The lunatic attendants refined themselves under the supervision of experienced attendants, the control of the house owners, the doctors and the visitors. The nature of this process of refinement was later reinforced, by the inclusion of the Board of Control and different Lunatic Acts of Parliament, together with experience of the attendants' skill, by Connelly, who delivered a set of lectures in relation to practice. The tension between personal experience, knowledge, social control and the control of education had started. Relating theory to practice and personal experience became such a tension up until the present time.

This experiential approach and the tensions created by it will form the basis of addressing the issues raised by the accounts of the students' educational experiences in this section, the experience of training being the main focus of the thesis. The report of the research comprises the following:

- a description of how the research started and developed, and the groups of students who took part in it;
- an account of the training syllabuses and the clinical environment for training;
- an outline of the students' backgrounds;
- an account of the form of presentation of the data: the historical link with the main categories and how they coordinated with the subcategories drawn from the students' list of statements;
- a presentation of students' accounts along with commentaries and a summary for each category. The summaries will point out the tensions inherent in the students' accounts, and this issue will be addressed in Section III.

Chapter 6
Method and presentation of data

How the research started and developed and the students who took part in it

The research started with a group of students registered for mental nursing courses who were expressing their concerns and anxieties to me about how they were experiencing their training. Their concerns centred around the problem of how to use their experiences and knowledge in clinical situations, this issue being a constant preoccupation of their training. In addition to this, many psychiatric hospitals were from this time onwards to close, and future student groups' documents of training were rewritten to meet the needs of the twenty-first century. Students were concerned about getting employment because of the effect of hospital closure and about their ability to carry out their responsibilities as a staff nurse once qualified. This made them feel let down and despondent as they felt that their course and training had been undervalued because the new document of training carried the Registered Mental Nurse as well as a Diploma in Health Studies qualification.

This group of students took an active part in a research project on the process of change, which I undertook for a Master's course, being concerned about the changes and the effect on students. From the start, the students wanted to be heard and to relate their accounts. My early interest was in cultural relativism and mental health. At that time, I was developing my interest in phenomenology, and history has always appealed.

Taking the students' and my own concerns into account, I expressed my interest in a research project. The students invited six students from the previous group who were prepared to take part. They made it clear that they wanted to speak from a student perspective of how they experienced their training. The first meeting consisted of 18 student nurses. Their aim was to have a group discussion on issues that were of

61

interest to them in relation to the school and their clinical placements, where they gained practical skills. We produced five A3 sheets and a blackboard full of ideas within the first 3 hours. These lists were then narrowed down to a list of 22 statements, as follows:

1. The role of experience in the negotiation of training.
2. How can you relate your experience to the plan of training to come out with a syllabus that is negotiable?
3. The use of experiential learning can bridge the gap between theory and practice.
4. Self-assertion in the classroom/ward.
5. Is nursing being thrown in at the deep end?
6. The position of the student nurse in relation to other professionals.
7. Subgrouping at a clinical level.
8. The anxiety/fear associated with training.
9. Evaluation by peers/others.
10. Past experience in education and its effects on you now.
11. The importance of the student nurse support group.
12. Mentors and supervision.
13. Finance – social position and rewards.
14. Roles and identity during training.
15. Do the 3 years influence my interaction with others?
16. Responsibility as a student.
17. The effects of clients on my developments.
18. The importance of projects/lectures.
19. The relationship between student nurse and management.
20. Is self-direction too demanding?
21. Allocation and relationship (clinical placements).
22. Ground rules and safety during training.

The other groups of students who took part in the research agreed to the above statements as long as they could interpret the statements to meet their purposes.

The views expressed by the initial discussion group was that the list had been narrowed down too much: they wanted it to be used as a checklist for discussions. However, another view expressed was that individuals should take what concerned them as a guide to express their feelings. At the end, the following format was agreed:

- Using the list of statements to describe the students' experiences in writing, based on individual accounts, with no limit set on the amount to be written.

- Using the list of statements to hold group discussions, which were to be recorded on audiotape.
- Using the part of the list relevant to individuals to give their account.
- For one group who took part in the research, the October 88 group, deciding that they should be able to use their own intuition, which meant dividing the list of topics between them, to be used to relate their experiences over a period of 6 months. This was to be followed by a presentation to the group and a group discussion.

The list was completed, but the project presented some hurdles in that permission had to be obtained from the Director of Nurse Education before the research could start. The conditions set were:

- I had to give a presentation of what I intended to do to a group of senior nurse tutors, justifying what the research was about, the method of research to be used and the groups I intended to use for the research.
- I was requested to produce an account of 3000 words detailing what the research would be about and the time I expected to spend on the project.
- The research should not interfere with the teaching load and student supervision.
- The time to be allocated for the research was 3 hours per week, and I was not to use the school's facilities.

The students who took part in the research decided to do so in their own time. The nursing school, part of the college or university, did not then support research students for a PhD, the course being self-financed. The past year has seen the provision of more support in that I have been given one full day a week study time and the possibility of financial assistance to complete the research.

One hundred and thirteen lists of statements (questionnaires) were sent out. The groups who took part were:

- intakes drawn from students registering in: May 87, September 87, May 88, October 88, September 90, March 93 and September 94 (Table 6.1);
- four qualified staff.

The above groups volunteered to take part in the research once they were made aware of the project by the students who were taking part. They were also requested to participate in the work by their personal

Table 6.1: Groups of students taking part in the research

82 syllabus group	Branch	Sites
May 87	Mental health	In the North
September 87	Mental health	In the North
May 88	Mental health	In the North
October 88	Mental health	In the North
Project 2000		
September 90	Mental health	Six clinical placements from three northern counties
March 93	Mental health	Six clinical placements from three northern counties
September 94	Mental health	Six clinical placements from three northern counties

The names of the sites have been withheld to prevent identification.

tutor and myself. The characteristics of the groups are shown in Table 6.2, and the response rate and details of questions not answered in Tables 6.3 and 6.4.

The written data, in the form of individual accounts, were completed by the members of the above groups. In the group of May 87, two students gave a joint account for statements 1 and 2. In the May 88 group, three students answered the 22 statements jointly after holding discussions among themselves; these three were BAC, LO and LA In the group starting in October 88, three students wrote in their own style, which was not directly related to the list. The number of students who took part in writing the individual accounts was 86 in total. The individual accounts ranged from three A4 sheets to 25 sheets. There was no limit set on how much information could be given.

The students who took part in the discussion groups were from the May 87, May 88 and October 88 groups. Each group took part in three 1-hour discussions and were audiotape-recorded. There were 40 students across the three groups.

The research was thus developed along these lines, the ways in which students wished to participate influencing the methodology to be used. Information was gathered from different sources, from personal accounts in relation to training, from recorded group discussions, from individual accounts of training over a 6-month clinical experience and from subgroup discussions. This style of research, in which participants can express their views in ways which they perceive to be appropriate, lies clearly within the qualitative research tradition, in particular

Table 6.2: The range of age and sex distribution in each group

Age group	May 87	Sept 87	May 88	Oct 88	Sept 90	Mar 93	Sept 94
18–25		12				9	20
25–35	4	4			2	4	6
35–45	7	2				3	5
45–55	1				1	4	1
No. of males	7	6	5	6	2	8	8
No. of females	5	12	7	4	1	12	24

Table 6.3: Response to statements

Group	No. of students	No. sent out	Response rate	Not answered
May 87	12	12	9	3
September 87	18	18	16	2
May 88	12	12	8	4
October 88	16	16	16	0
September 90	20	3	3	0
March 93	20	20	14	6
September 94	32	32	22	10
Total	130	113	88	25

The total number of statements/questions distributed between May 1990 and October 1992, and April and August 1997, was 130; in addition, 4 more went to qualified staff.

within phenomenology, the lived experience of the students (Merleau-Ponty 1962) and the grounded theory of Strauss & Corbin (1990). In phenomenology, methodology is aimed at eliciting participants' perspectives without prior conceptualization, and in grounded theory the intention is to allow general formulations to arise from the data. I have not therefore attempted a numerical qualification of the data in presenting students' views but have attempted to show these through the students' typical and atypical responses.

The training syllabuses and the clinical environment for training

In the research carried out for this thesis, there were two styles of training running parallel to each other, both converging in that they were taught by the same teaching staff, offered a similar experience in clinical situations and were supervised by the same clinician/mentor.

Table 6.4: Number of students in the group who did not answer the appropriate statement

Statement No.	May 87	Sept 87	May 88	Oct 88	Sept 90	Mar 93	Sept 94
1		2			1		
2							2
3		2	1				1
4	1						
5			1				
6			1				
7							2
8							
9	1	1					3
10							1
11							1
12							1
13			2				1
14			1				1
15			1				2
16		2	1			1	2
17		2	1			1	1
18			1			1	3
19	1	1				1	1
20	1					1	2
21	5	7	3	1		2	3
22	4	8	2	1		1	3

The training documents/syllabuses of the two were different, but there was a similarity in the content taught. The two courses were the 82 syllabus, which started in 1986 (it was called the 82 syllabus because the recommendation for that style of training was made by the Nursing Council in 1982, although it was not implemented until the middle 1980s) and Project 2000, which was approved by 1990. The content of the Project 2000 syllabus differs in that it was arranged in subject areas based on social sciences and nursing theories – psychology, sociology, biological science, nursing models and ethics – whereas in the 82 syllabus, though these subjects were covered, they were integrated. The 82 syllabus spent a third of the training studying theoretical perspective and two-thirds in clinical practice, whereas the Project 2000 syllabus was 50% theory and 50% practice.

The training for the 82 syllabus group was a block of 15 weeks in college followed by a community project, which had to be presented to the students' tutor group, the 3 years' training being in mental health placements, with one module in a physical care area. Each module was an 8–12-week placement in a particular clinical area with a preparation block and a feedback study block at the beginning and end respectively. A 3-week self-directed study block, as well as an elective placement for 3 weeks, was allocated during the second year. The purpose of the elective placement was for the students to develop an area of interest, which could be either local, national or international. This group had to take a state examination as well as achieving the required level of clinical skills as laid down by the English National Board.

Clinical placements for 82 syllabus were in the following areas:

- acute care
- general nursing
- elderly care (organic disorders)
- elderly care (functional disorders)
- community care
- a rehabilitation unit
- specialist care
- a management unit.

For Project 2000 groups, the course was organized in units, the first 18 months being an introduction to social sciences, biological sciences and nursing models. This first part had to be undertaken by every student nurse. It consisted of 22 weeks of theory in the college/university followed by a placement of 4 weeks in a specialist area of nursing, for example the mental health, adult nursing, child, midwifery or learning disabilities branch. The placement was followed by a non-institutional community placement (meaning not hospital based), at the end of which the students had to present a locality study and a special interest study.

The theoretical assessment in the first 18 months (the Common Foundation Programme or CFP) consisted of two examinations: one seen and one unseen paper. Students also had to write two projects of 2500 words each. At the end of the CFP, there is a transition unit to the branch of interest. The mental health branch, which is the concern of this project, consisted of unit six, unit seven (an elective placement) and units eight and nine, which are classified as 'rostered duty', meaning that students had to be seen as members of staff on the placement for 1000 hours. This placement is seen as skill based and fostering the learning necessary to become a qualified nurse. It is followed by unit ten, a 4-week management unit. During this time, the 18-month mental health branch, there are three theoretical assignments of 2500 words, with a seen paper examination.

The training syllabuses for both of the courses were based on a spiral curriculum approach. It was stated to the students that the courses would be self-directed. The objectives for each unit were stated, albeit in a somewhat repetitive fashion. The students were expected to use their experiences in the project work and written examinations. The documents did not direct how these should be done, the process being left to individual tutor's group. The examinations and projects were monitored by external examiners who were teaching members of higher education from other institutions. In both courses, the 82 syllabus and the Project 2000 students had to achieve the required level of clinical competencies at different levels of training. This was supervised and monitored by the supervisor/mentor, the nursing lecturers and the examination committee. Not achieving the required level might lead to a delay in registration. The Project 2000 students were, at the end of the 3 years' training, registered with the UKCC as registered mental nurses, as well as being awarded a diploma in nursing studies.

The mental health branch placements for Project 2000 were:

- acute care
- elderly care
- community care
- a continuing care/rehabilitation unit
- acute care/management.

These courses are held on different sites. The 82 syllabus groups were site specific; the Project 2000 students completed the CFP in the selected sites and then joined the mental health branch, which was made up of the mental health team in the Mental Health and Learning Disabilities Nursing Department. The teaching took place in one site, the clinical placements being situated in the area that the student had selected prior to training. The areas were clinical sites in six towns or cities in three different counties, with a radius averaging 55 miles.

These sites formed part of the faculty of medicine within the university in the North. The facilities on the sites had lending libraries, with the exception of one of the sites in the central part (now closed), which had only a reference library. These students had to use libraries within the medical schools in the north and south of the city as well as the main university library. The individual site libraries could be used by any students of the university, each library also being equipped with CD-roms and catalogues to which the students could gain access.

The clinical environments comprised the psychiatric services in these three northern counties; voluntary agencies, specialist psychiatric organizations, local authority facilities and some private inpatient establishments were also utilized for clinical experiences. The clinical circuits were monitored regularly on a yearly or 6-monthly basis by nursing lecturers, who were, with the assistance of the clinicians, responsible for quality control. The nursing lecturers were also responsible for making regular visits to their specified areas to keep clinicians informed of any educational policy changes.

The clinical staff who were responsible for supervising or mentoring students were all qualified mental health nurses with at least 6 months' post-registered experience as a staff nurse. It was recommended that they take a teaching and assessors course as part of their development to become supervisors. They were responsible for completing the practical assessment documents of students under their supervision.

The mental health placements were still being influenced by the closure of different sites and the movement into community care. This movement started in the early 1980s, the effect of the change still influencing students and staff as this affected their employment prospects and choice of clinical placement for experience. It was in the midst of this change process, which was influencing the placement, and the change from the syllabus to Project 2000, that I developed an interest in this research.

The thesis addressed the relevance of experience to practice. Although the students who took part were from two different syllabuses, my intention is not to show the differences between the two courses. After presenting the data, I will make some remarks on this issue.

An outline of the student groups' background

The groups were of mixed educational background, ranging across the following (Table 6.5):

- graduates in social sciences;
- a teacher with teaching qualifications;
- those with GCE 'O' Level, 'A' Level and GCSE grades 2 or 3;
- a student with a BTec National Diploma (although this student left training withing 3 three months);
- an NVQ qualification;
- a DC Test – an aptitude test devised by Denise Child, Professor of Education at the University of Newcastle;
- nursing experience as a State Enrolled Nurse (SEN);
- unqualified nursing backgrounds, ranging from 6 months to 15 years in nursing.

Table 6.5: Educational background of the students

Group	Graduate	Cert Ed	GCE/GCSE	SEN	DC	BTec
May 87	0	0	8	1	3	0
September 87	3	0	13	0	2	0
May 88	1	1	6	1	3	0
October 88	4	0	10	0	2	0
September 90	1	0	14	0	5	0
March 93	3	0	13	0	4	0
September 94	2	0	26	0	4	0

The presentation of the data as categories and subcategories

The data will be presented into two parts. The first of these, the individual accounts (Chapter 7), will present the individual experiences of 86 students by presenting the accounts they gave directed by the checklist of statements.

The second part, group discussions and student reflections (Chapter 8), will be presented as commentaries of the recorded discussions of May 87 (12 students), May 88 (12 students) and October 88 (2 of the students). One personal account presented in the original work has been omitted (see Ramsamy 1998).

The presentation of this data will take the historical perspective into account. From the historical study of the caring aspect (Section I), we have seen how madness was managed in relation to different social contexts. Prior to the institutionalization of madness, and even during the earlier days of this institutionalization, experiencing madness and recovering from it was a way to help others in their despair. Up to and during the time of Tuke, the way in which acute patients used their experience to develop the role of attendant became clearer. Matrons, housekeepers and 'visitors' were encouraged on a Sunday to show attendants how to behave. By imitating the visitors, they would therefore be able to display the same behaviour, and this would then influence the patients in their interactions with others. The process of learning through supervision and imitation thus started, the role of the manager/matron being introduced in this manner.

We saw that in France, historically, caring often involved a conflict between the junior medical staff and experienced sisters, whereas in India the power of the mentor to guide a person through stress and the co-ordination of self-development was emphasized (see Section I). The institutionalization of madness also brought with it an element of control, not only of the mad, but also of the attendants. The control was initially effected through the institution itself, the Lunatic Acts and Mental Health Act, but nowadays the control of mental health nurses lies with the UKCC, the legal system and terms of employment. With this element of control and the institutionalization of carers, care became relocated, and the conflict of financial interest/wage for care became a constant social and economic struggle.

Bringing madness and carers into a system of control moved the system of training away from that of experiencing madness, being cared for with supervision and learning by imitation. This system was perceived to be inadequate as the scientific gaze, in the form of the medical model, penetrated the management of madness and caring. In coping with this, Connelly (1856) was the first to start lecturing on madness and to relate it to clinical situations. This was in effect the birth of reflective practice since mental health nursing was required to relate theory to practice through a reference to clinical situations.

It was on the basis of this account, and on a close analysis of the 22 statements, that it became apparent that six main categories could summarize the concerns of those involved in mental health care and training, both now and historically. These six main categories are:

1. The relevance of experience to training
2. Theory and practice: how do students bridge the gap?
3. The role of mentorship/supervision: how do students learn within this mode?
4. Learning in the clinical setting: how do students relate to the real-life learning environment?
5. How do students perceive their relationship with others in clinical settings?
6. What effects does training have on the students?

The list of 22 statements that guided the research are arranged as subcategories under these six main headings. Historically, these six categories have their place in the attendants' style of training. Similar issues seem to repeat themselves in the learning climate today, creating various tensions and concerns in mental health nurse training.

The conflicts, continuities and contradictions of care are contained in the accounts or reports of the students' lived experience of training. We shall see that the medical framework still influenced their experiences, especially in the main categories 4 and 5, which deal with learning in the clinical setting and how students perceive their relationship with others in this setting.

Table 6.6 shows the list of 22 statements in relation to the six categories.

Table 6.6: Categories and subcategories* used in the research

Subcategories	Relationship with statement no.
1. The relevance of experience to training	
a. The role of experience in the negotiation of training	1
b. Is nursing being thrown in at the deep end?	5
c. Past experience in education and its effects on you now	10
d. Does the three years influence my interaction with others?	15
2. Theory and practice: how do students bridge the gap?	
a. How they relate their experience to a plan of training, to come out with a syllabus that is negotiable	2
b. The use of experiential learning to bridge the gap between theory and practice	3
c. The effects of the client on my development	17
d. The importance of projects and lectures	18
3. The role of mentorship/supervision: how do students learn within this mode?	
a. Evaluation by peers and others	9
b. Mentorship and supervision	12
c. Role and identity during training	14
4. Learning in the clinical setting: how the students relate to the real-life learning environment	
a. The position of the student nurse in relation to other professionals, as perceived by the students	6
b. Is self-direction too demanding?	20
c. Allocation and relationships with others in the clinical setting	21
5. How do students perceive their relationship with others in clinical settings?	
a. Subgrouping at clinical level	7
b. The importance of the student nurse support group	11
c. Responsibility as a student	16
d. The relationship between student nurse and management	19
6. What effects does training have on the students?	
a. Self-assertion in the classroom/ward	4
b. Anxiety/fear associated with training	8
c. Finance/social position and reward	13
d. Ground rules and safety during training	22

*Fitting the statements into the subcategories was an extremely difficult task; 1(d), for example, could also appear in 6.

These categories and subcategories interlink with each other, as will become obvious in the next chapter. The way in which they interreact and create tensions was apparent through history; in the French perspective, for example, the conflict between the junior doctors and the sisters could be seen as affecting the relationship in clinical settings and the role of the mentor during training.

An alphabetical code is used in order to retain the confidentiality of the students who took part: for XH/C.82.S, XH denotes the initials of the student pseudoname, C the month in which the course started and 82.S or K2.S the syllabus followed by the group. The year, for example 87 or 93, has been omitted to minimize the risk of identification of the participants. This coding system will be used throughout the book when referring to the data and for the presentation of data in the following chapters.

Chapter 7
Individual accounts

Category 1: The relevance of experience to training

This category is made up of the four following subcategories under which the accounts will be related:

a. The role of experience in the negotiation of training
b. Is nursing being thrown in at the deep end?
c. Past experience in education and its effects on you now
d. Does the three years influence my interaction with others?

Subcategory 1a

A significant number of students expressed the view that the opportunity to negotiate came too early during their training. They felt that they could not negotiate on something they knew very little about. Negotiation was seen as 'go and find out for yourself':

> A certain amount of flexibility in training, i.e. options of which wards to work on, I have found valuable in both motivating myself and being allowed to gain experience in areas I am interested in. However, at first psychiatric nursing was to me a totally unknown quantity. I knew nothing about it so when confronted with the 'well what do you want to do' statement, I started to feel anger and resentment towards the School as I felt that they should have 'all the answers' and they should be directing me the way they think best. This responsibility at such an early stage of my training made me feel quite insecure and unskilled. So, yes, I feel some form of negotiation is very valuable, but I did not realize quite how valuable until the latter part of my training, i.e. third year, maybe end of second. At first I feel I would have gained more benefit from a more rigid structure up to the end of the first year, perhaps especially the introduction block. (MX/C.82.S)

There was a certain amount of negotiation available, especially in the Common Foundation Programme. However, there were many 'unforeseen' items occurring which tended to make it hard to make plans. Self-directed study time is good in theory up to a point; however, it came at such a time that we were unable to make the most of it as at this time we were unsure where our priorities should be. (BX/T.K2.S)

A proportion of students also expressed the view that they needed guidance for their experience to be meaningful and that the institution was not really prepared for meaningful negotiation:

Student nurses are and should be encouraged to have a high degree of input into negotiating their training. To what degree this negotiation has any real effect on the direction of training I am unsure. It is my feeling that the syllabus of training will be adhered to by most tutors despite any input from students. In many respects this is fair as from my own experience I needed guidance from my tutor, but I also needed respect as a person, which was given. This I feel is the exception, not the rule. (FX/C.82.S)

I think it is very difficult to plan anything without any experience or understanding of the matter involved. Though prior to entering nursing we all have experience of our own mental health and that of family, friends, etc., 'the Health Service' is something other. The mechanisms and philosophies of the system need to be experienced to some degree before an idea of what is wanted can be found and then negotiated. Even then negotiation is very difficult unless the service is run on lines of negotiation, discussion, mutual respect. Unfortunately Sheffield has too many children of the institution in power who seem unable to adapt to a more open approach. (ON/C.82.S)

There were 17 students who expressed the need for tutorial support and the importance of coordination between clinical staff, students and teaching staff in the structuring and processing of training. Many of them had not experienced any form of self-directed learning:

At the outset of the course, particularly introductory block, it was emphasized quite strongly that the learning content of the course (i.e. school study) could be (and perhaps even should be) directed by the group. This however did not seem to happen possibly for a couple of reasons.

1. It appeared that people in the group, including myself, were looking for direction from course leaders (many of us had never

experienced self-directed learning styles), and we complained that we did not know how to organize the course as we did not know what we were supposed to be learning and what the options were.

2. There was no strong leader in the group to take the initiative in suggesting course direction for the others to follow.
3. Certain tutors, although stating that the group should direct its own course, did not seem totally comfortable with the learner-centred approach or with giving up power to the group. Some suggestions that were made did not meet the approval of the tutor, and sometimes inadequate explanations were given as to why these ideas were unsuitable. This made me and others cynical as to how much say we really did have.
4. Tutors changed frequently; some encouraged negotiation, others were directive, often leaving the group floundering.

I'm still in some confusion as to the degree we can plan our training, particularly clinical placements. For the first year to 15 months we all went to areas that were allocated to us, and it seemed that the only choice that could be exercised was during our elective placement. However, since then certain more assertive members of the group have been requesting where they go on their allocations. There does not seem to be any clear guidelines about this. The School of Nursing seems to be quietly allowing certain people a degree of choice in where they go but not broadcasting it too loudly, presumably to prevent everyone asserting their choice, which will add to the present adminis-tration problems. (XI/C.82.S)

The responsibility of negotiating must be with the group's tutor, so a tutor who knows and understands individuals in the group is essen-tial. When students negotiate allocations, etc. with staff outside the School of Nursing, this still needs supervision of a tutor to provide infor-mation and ensure agreed objectives are adhered to. (YT/D.82.S)

Thirteen of the students valued the experience retrospectively, although they found it intimidating and frustrating at first. Here are two examples:

There were times when I found it quite frustrating that I was not told what to do and what to learn but instead was given space and time and asked to decide how to use it. However, I did not have to wait too long to see how this could lead to a group of people looking at issues which were important to them and learning through this system. The lessons learnt were more meaningful because they were not presented to us by

a teacher from a syllabus but were what we had decided to ask.
(UG/C.82.S)

In my experience there are a few areas in which I feel that I was not
a participant in negotiations. Firstly, within the group certain dominant
members of the group appeared to railroad the more meek and mild
members of the group, who were less confident in themselves, such as
myself, so that I followed some discussions and roads which I felt at the
time were inappropriate and not really related to the job I was training
for. Now I realize that some areas were connected, but at the time that
we approached them they seemed inappropriate. Also some areas
were of no real interest to me. When a firmer grip was taken on the
plan of training and also when I developed my confidence and felt
more able to join in the negotiation, I felt that the plan of training was
more to my 'liking'. Perhaps this was selfish, but by this time I was angry
that I had always had to consider others' needs before my own and felt
that my needs were now more important to me than other people due
to the way these people had treated me. (BG/C.82.S)

Ten of the students felt they could not take part in negotiating their
training due to timetable restrictions:

Student nurses can plan their training during a placement but not in
block. (MX/T.K2.S)

To a limited degree, i.e. non-clinical placements, community placements – otherwise academic requirements appear to be structured/
non-negotiable. (FX/T.K2.S)

One student felt there was a lack of resources, meaning clinical
placements for experience, and a shortage of teaching staff:

The choices are not completely free, being limited by POLITICAL obsta-
cles related to resource thence to government funding, e.g. shortage of
clinical allocations to pick from, competition with numerous other
students (including the questionable debarring of RMN students from
P2000 wards/units, SHORTAGE OF FACILITATION AND GUIDANCE
TIME FROM TUTORS, because tutors themselves are under-strength.
(IT/D.82.S)

A group of 10 students felt that they needed practical experience in
the field prior to any form of negotiation. This view was shared by a
majority of those who had been care assistants before starting their
training:

The question which was put forward [was] 'Can SEN plan their training with negotiation?'; from the beginning I would say no, a certain amount of guidance and direction is needed as many like myself came into RMN not knowing what to expect or what there is available, resources and sources that are there. Perhaps at 18 months when various wards have been covered, along with the theoretical work, one may know which direction one wants to move in, and then if possible should be able to plan the following 18 months, but whether or not it is realistic in assuming that nurse education would agree with this ...

I can remember the first week in School and it was put to the group, it was up to us to plan what we wanted to do within that week. It brought to me a sense of panic, confusion, how was one expected to put suggestions forward if we didn't know what the course entailed. Previous training, SEN, was a directed approach learning systematically bodily functions and the disease process which may affect that system and treatment and nursing management of that disease, with little emphasis on the client, their thoughts and feelings. It felt as though I had been thrown into a alien environment, not knowing how to react or what to expect; it was alien enough having to sit within a group of strangers and telling these strangers a little about yourself, without having the added confusion of 'what do you want to do?' (C./S.82.S)

I entered nursing with a very clear idea of what I wanted from my 3 years training – which skills and experiences I wished to acquire. This is because I had already spent 3.5 years as a nursing assistant on acute wards.

Students beginning their training have varying degrees of nursing experience and consequently varying ideas of what they want from their training. Most learners probably do not have a clear idea of where they want to do until they are at least 18 months/2 years into their training. (BW/S.82.S)

A proportion of students felt that the objectives for the course and the conditions for placements were set before the course started. This created a feeling of being limited when it came to negotiating:

From the onset of the 3 year RMN course the aims and objectives of the group (individuals) were clearly set out in the ENB 1982 syllabus. Outlining the course the training would follow, i.e. practical experience, the nurse could negotiate where she could spend her speciality, but within limitations, and professional development was negotiated again with limitations as one could not go on a ward which the Project 2000 nurses were training. (CC/S.82.S)

In an ideal world there is scope for student nurses to plan their training with negotiations as long as the negotiation phase employs guidance as to the appropriateness of which areas are followed and the legal and other restrictions placed by the ENB, School of Nursing, etc. (BG/S.82.S)

Summary of subcategory 1a

The individual accounts of the students gave a clear view that there is a need for practical experience in caring for those with mental health problems, together with appropriate guidance, before the students can take part in the negotiation of their training. This view was supported by a majority of the students, being backed up by the accounts of those students who completed the 2 years' training (SEN) and supported by those who were care assistants before they started the RMN course.

A large proportion of the students called for an improvement in the coordination between teaching staff, clinical staff and students. These students also made the point that they wanted a tutor who knew them personally to take part in this coordination. The majority of the students expressed the view that they wanted to be directed by a leadership to whom they could explain their needs. Some of the accounts portrayed the documents of training and the timetables as not allowing the space for negotiation and argued that negotiations can take place only in clinical allocations where they could gain experience. Most of the students supported the view that negotiation could only take place during the last year of training. Only one student saw the lack of resources as a problem in the negotiating of training needs.

The comments made showed mixed feelings. Some viewed their previous experiences as being so limited that they needed a lot of support or guidance to negotiate in a meaningful way. The opportunity to negotiate created conflicting feelings of fear, excitement and vulnerability; the directive approach to teaching they had experienced in the past created a felt demand to meet objectives, and this was seen as inhibiting successful negotiating early in the course. A fair proportion found the training to be marred by legal restrictions and constraints from the UKCC and English National Board for Nursing, Midwifery and Health Visiting (ENB), as well as by constraints on clinical placements caused by a shortage of facilities.

The views expressed by the students raised some issues relating to the process of training in relation to mental health care. The following two questions are noteworthy here, although I shall return to a fuller discussion at the end of Section II:

1. In view of the students' comments, should the course start with supervised practice in mental health care followed by theoretical input from the teaching staff?
2. Also, should there be a closer link between practice and theory and more attention given to this issue by the teaching staff?

Subcategory 1b

A majority of the 49 students expressed the feeling of being unprepared, the reasons being the gaps in communication between teaching staff and a lack of preparation by the school of students for clinical placements. The students felt that the theoretical framework provided was too superficial to be meaningful in practice:

> Traditionally, as far as I understand, nursing training has consisted of a ward apprenticeship – being thrown into the task of running and managing a ward environment. In my opinion this mentality still prevails. My experience of the first few months of training was that the gap between School and ward is too wide for there to be any sense of gaining a knowledge base which can then be applied in the clinical setting. This seemed to come about for two reasons: (a) the initial experience in School was one of being thrown a smattering of superficial psychology, self-awareness exercises with an underlying sense that you'll start to learn something when you're on the ward; (b) once on the ward I found the main preoccupations of staff to be with management of clients on the ward, and any educational commitment to students (apart from basics of physical care) was seen as the responsibility of School. So, yes, I do feel nursing training still consists of being thrown in the deep end. (BX/D.82.S)
>
> Yes it is, especially in the first year. Experiential learning can only be supported by the established foundation of a theoretical framework. Without a meaningful knowledge base much of the first year allocations equate to being a 'tea boy'. It is an apprentice-like ritual that one must do one's general allocation early in the training. For me this was like being a fish out of water. My role was defined by token jobs – learning the trade. Much of the time in early allocations I felt redundant, bored and inferior. More time has to be spent on theory before being booted out onto wards! (SX/D.82.S)

One student thought that the course's emphasis on self-direction inhibited the development of appropriate skills:

> I would say, by the very nature of this course, with its emphasis on self-direction, it is not equipping nurses with the skills they require. It is all

too easy to complete this course without having given an injection, for example. Nurses are not being prepared with enough basic knowledge. In an ideal world our course would be wonderful, but we are not living in an ideal world and we cannot pick and choose what we would like to do. At the end of the day it is what is acceptable to the public. It does not help to improve one's status or help one to be assertive if you know about complicated theories but yet you cannot deliver an injection or know what the side-effects of the drug being administered are. It is easy to say you can gain help from other professionals, but having to ask them simple questions which they probably covered in the early stages of their training does not help the student gain status or respect, no matter how much theoretical knowledge they possess. (BC/N.K2.S)

Twenty-nine students argued that accepting responsibility for one's learning under support and supervision was a form of learning essential to the course, for example:

Yes, you cannot prescribe situations on the ward. It is 'the nature of the beast'. But being thrown in the deep end varies in seriousness between whether someone is standing on the side with a life-line or not! (LX/S.82.S)
    If this question means, are student nurses left to their own devices and made to fend for themselves?, then yes, to a certain degree I think this is true. Then again it depends where you are. In some instances the staff on the wards can be very supportive and appreciate the needs of students; on other areas they seem to resent the inconvenience. (BG/S.82.S)
    It can be a lot of time. Often you need to be thrown in at the deep end in order to grasp learning opportunities. If supervised properly this can be a beneficial experience. (WX/T.K2.S)

The following two students felt adequately prepared for their clinical experiences. This view was shared by a minority, mostly the mature age group:

My nurse training was not wholly sink or swim, although it was in many ways a test of the individual's ability to work alone or be extremely adaptive finding one allocation and its culture very different from another. The ability to adapt to changing environments and remain true to oneself is essential for mental health. (HX/S.82.S)
    I have not experienced this. I think students have very little real responsibility at first and this only increases at the rate students let it.

Common sense, rather than knowledge and understanding, is what is needed at the earlier stages of training. I have throughout the course found supervisors, etc. to be very good at only expecting of me what they know I am capable of doing. I believe it is necessary to be on a ward from early on in training (personally I found a 12-week intro block too long) as I think to get real grip of the theory one needs to see its application, and as demands are not too great, this can be done in comfort. (GF/T.82.S)

This student expressed the view that being introduced to the routine of the ward would help her to cope with situations:

After the initial 12 weeks in School you are basically thrown in at the deep end. I was left on my first ward to my own devices, the ward manager did not introduce herself or welcome me to the ward. I was not shown any of the daily routines, e.g. laundry, etc., and although this is not one of the major responsibilities, it is knowing the day-to-day running and small things that need to be done daily that helps students settle onto a ward quickly. It was never negotiated with me how the ward and I were to organize time with clients, and looking back, the ward really just bungled along with no fresh ideas and no philosophy except give the drugs out at drug time. I was expected to 'special' after about 3 days on the ward, not really being told what this was about or anything about the client to be specialized. (WP/C.82.S)

The two students quoted below identified the lack of resources as being an issue in caring and learning situations:

I feel nursing is suffering very badly from the present political situation. My opinion is, though, that the standard of nursing care has not fallen as quickly as the withdrawal of resources from nursing. This is because nurses appear to react in a time of adversity and work harder to cushion the effects. While this is admirable I feel it is political folly. (UG/C.82.S)

If by deep end you mean the clinical area, then yes as a student you are thrown in at the deep end. If resources could be used to provide students with supernumerary status, and resources in School brought to bear to provide better support with perhaps more study days in School, then maybe students could at least be provided with water wings. (CF/N.82.S)

One student considered confidentiality to be a major factor:

Throughout the three years training the School of Nursing professed to promote certain basic principles relevant to psychiatric nursing. One of these was confidentiality. Yet there was one occasion where the School itself actually breached confidentiality. This happened when a tutor (not the group's usual tutor) sat in with the group and I shared a personal experience. I fully expected that what I had said would remain confidential but the tutor shared it with others outside the group and practically said that I was 'mentally ill'. If the School of Nursing is capable of setting this example, it does not seem logical that it should be preaching what it does not appear to be practising. (RK/C.82.S)

Summary of subcategory 1b

A large number of students expressed the view that the gap between the clinical situations and what was taught in the School was too wide. In some cases, they believed that clinicians did not understand their needs. One of the major issues was that they were not prepared to cope with the skills needed on clinical placement, nor were they taught the skills required. Without these skills, these students felt that they had little confidence in the role they were asked to perform.

On the other hand, the majority of students expressed the point that the situation of being thrown in was in the nature of mental health nursing as clinical situations were often crisis situations. The major facilitating factors identified were clinical supervision and support, and the time to reflect on their experiences; these were their concerns in relation to how to develop skills, cope with clinical situations and changing environments as well as manage different clients during placements. The changing environment and having to work on their own were factors that helped some students to develop their individuality and others to feel inferior and unable to cope.

Three students identified clinical resources, staff levels and study time as their major concerns. One saw the breach of confidentiality as being of great importance, and another identified the introduction to the daily anxieties and ward routines as a way of being accepted and being able to cope.

What had been expressed by the students raised the following questions:

1. What should students be taught to prepare them for practice?
2. How should the supervision and the support of students be organized in order to facilitate learning at the clinical level?
3. Should theory follow practice and reflection?

Subcategory 1c

The minority of students, those who undertook a further or higher education course before starting nurse training, found their experiences, especially the study skills, useful:

> My academic (degree) experience has been of great use to me – my ability to read fast, research, etc., write – though not directly related to nursing; I feel any further education can be made use of in learning skills, experience, ability to take in knowledge. The disadvantage is that I am easily bored when things get too slow in School and switch off, feeling a bit of an academic snob. The other advantage of having had further education is an appreciation of being a student again and being in a learning environment. (MX/D.82.S)
> I found doing 'A' levels before the course a great help with assignments and course work. (WK/S.K2.S)

Some students pointed out that a teacher-led style of teaching made it difficult for them to work in small groups and be assertive:

> Has made me think in very concrete terms – black and white. Studied science-based subjects – not encouraged to think/explore for myself. Just had to learn information 'parrot-fashion' for exams. Find nursing exams difficult as a result. Learning within a group has been very difficult (alien) for me – after 20 years of sitting behind desks! Very challenging – still haven't completely mastered it. (BW/S.82.S)
> Both schooling primary and secondary and further training all took a directive approach. Sat behind tables, tutor at the front, following a rigid timetable. (RP/S.82.S)

These two students expressed the view that having a goal to work for motivated them:

> The difference between the education received at school then and that which I have now completed as a student nurse is that there has been a great deal of motivation and interest in the subject areas studied in comparison to that of secondary school. As a mature student the willingness and motivation has been directed towards a goal which tends to provide an impetus and drive. (MD/N.K2.S)
> I consider I had a very poor education and only really began to learn when I took the responsibility for this myself. After shaking off my negative attitude to my educative attainments, I have been able to 'use'

education for my own advantage – which I have used throughout the course. (AP/N.82.S)

The directive approach, the teacher-led style, made a majority of students feel guilty during nurse training. They were used to discipline that kept them motivated. In nursing, the self-directed approach created a problem for them, especially when they had to complete projects in a set time. Here is one example:

I look back with resentment at the fact that I was channelled into specific areas and learning in a specific way.

While self-directed learning is fine for one at 28, at 10 years I really didn't know what was good for me, as they say!!

I suppose that I am somewhat bitter about school and indeed will seek to prevent my own children from going through the same things.

I would have preferred (with hindsight) to have been allowed to learn experientially with some subtle guidance and direction given, e.g. this is the objective but there is no set route to meeting that objective.

This has made reading/research difficult. I still think 'Have I got my homework to do?' and feel guilty for doing nothing during the evening. I found I could commit myself to areas of true interest in academic work, but since my philosophy is far removed from study or academic then I could not really get into it. (RP/C.82.S)

Past experience in education left these students feeling depersonalized and dull:

Until my RMN I never felt personally involved in education. It is the only course I have experienced in which I applied principle and observation to self, myself, by first feeling and thought and later reflection in order to assess its worth and impact upon my concept of self and view of the universe. In this way, the 3 year course has been my first formal education in how to use and understand my life and the world of relationships around me. Prior to that, education had been a very dull process of passing on information, and unless the teacher or tutor had a personal love for their topic/subject, it was impersonal and unmoving – the opposite of my experience of RMN training. (JX/C.82.S)

Although my previous experiences of education have been marred by the depersonalization of the education system, the knowledge and experiences gained can be a useful resource to draw upon, both theoretically and in practice. (BT/N.82.S)

This one student was left affected by the competitive and negative aspect of the educational system:

> The downfall I believe to be is the way it takes no account of the individual nature of each student. Another negative aspect I feel is the use of competition to spur on individuals. This may be fine for the able students but those who are less able become 'losers' in the environment of competition.
>
> The first factor now has very little effect on me. I am aware of its downfalls and have managed to adopt the attitudes of looking for people's strengths.
>
> What has had a more lasting effect is the aspect of competition. While I am aware of how destructive competition can be, I have to be constantly wary to stop myself becoming competitive in everyday situations. (UG/C.82.S)

Some of the students felt that their past education was not relevant and they were left with feelings of being demotivated, whereas other small groups felt that their past education did not prepare them for the academic work they were undertaking in nursing. Here is one example of each case:

> I don't really feel that my past education has made really any relevance to things I have done and learnt on this course. From finishing school I took two years out, although does not sound long, I found it difficult to get into the habit of studying again. (BB/N.K2.S)
>
> I feel my past educational experience did not prepare me for the level of academic writing that has been required. I find this has been a challenge to come up to scratch. Also I now feel as though I would like to do further academic courses. (HY/N.K2.S)

Summary of subcategory 1c

A majority of the students felt that their past experience in education was teacher led. Whilst some felt that they benefited from the style of learning in that they were taught to carry out literature searches, interpret literature and work within small groups, this view was contradicted by a majority who felt that previous educational experience did not benefit them; they reported feelings of demotivation and feeling guilty for not doing their projects, of being dull and undisciplined in their work. One student commented upon the negative and competitive nature of his previous education. A small group felt that they started learning when they took responsibility for their education and were working towards a goal.

Overall, past education has left a significant number of the students with problems in working with small groups and in asserting themselves in group situations. It is thus evident that the style of learning demanded by nurse training is at odds with the previous experience of many students. This creates tensions, which any effective course should clearly be aware of.

Subcategory 1d

This one student perceived the wide experience as being blinkered. Psychiatric nurses were viewed as using a special stock of phraseology:

> I have found psychiatric nursing very incestuous, very easy to club together and ignore the people on the outside. Very easy to follow each other, very hard to be different. But I also found the same sort of relationships in the police force as I think there may be in any large institution. I found it very easy to get into the habit of working with nurses, living with nurses and socializing with nurses. This has a tendency to make one narrow-minded and blinkered, seeing outsiders as a threat. Nursing starts to affect your interactions with others in the way that you begin to analyse too deeply, look for things that aren't there and communicate using psychiatric nursing stock phrases and counselling techniques in an off the cuff and patronizing way. (WP/S.82.S)

These three students found their job affecting their social life, especially how they interacted with others:

> Yes, I don't usually tell people what my job is unless they specifically ask. I try not to take the job home or out socially with me. It is hard not to, but you need a break, especially when things are intense at work. (AW/D.82.S)
>
> Interaction outside of work – yes, the 'taking my work home' syndrome. Difficult to break off from goings on in work. Influences my approach to others in terms of confidence, self and other awareness, patient, rights, etc. I feel I am now more open to criticism and comment and other opinions and have learned a non-judgmental approach. (TB/D.82.S)
>
> Yes, I have found that most of the people I know are involved in one way or another in the health profession and don't seem to know anyone who is not. (AW/3.K2.S)

These two students expressed the opposite view from the above three, although they experienced a change in their level of self-confidence, self-assertion and interaction with others:

Broadly speaking, no. The training has increased interactive skills and assertiveness but this has come through experience which arguably could have come from other quarters. Perhaps I am more aware of how I interact with other people than before. Experiencing death at close hand has obvious implications for both professional and personal perspectives. (KG/D.82.S)

No, it doesn't influence me, not significantly. Perhaps significantly, I have not changed or adapted much in respect of my overall identity and overall behaviour during training (i.e. outside my 'on duty' role). Looking within the area of student nurse work here I do continue to develop/learn/self-study, e.g. on areas of personal, stress management, work load management, client interaction skills. (OI/D.82.S)

Losing the feeling of naivety or innocence during interaction was a consequence of training to the next student:

In social situations I think that I have lost a certain naivety or innocence which sometimes I do miss. I seem to spend more time examining my own feelings and those of others and dissecting social encounters after the event. Perhaps this is something I have always done but now I am armed with the labels and theories which mean I can make a seemingly clinical evaluation. (KK/N.82.S)

These two students found themselves becoming more critical towards their families, which led to a drop in their level of self-confidence:

Unfortunately yes! I have been criticized on occasion by both partner and family for sounding like 'a bloody nurse', rather than the partner/son/brother they are used to. Though I think I can justify what I have said I am equally quick to criticize others who I see as being full of 'academic ...' and not as down to earth as myself. This conflict is yet to be resolved.

I also feel increased awareness of self has led to a drop in confidence. I think I was happier being arrogant and ignorant but other people would probably prefer me to be more pleasant if a little shyer. (MX/D.82.S)

The course has had a profound influence on my life and all my relationships; at first losing some of my self confidence and to some extent my personality was distorted by a period of overinvolved group culture which thankfully has resolved itself with my adopting some of its aspects into an already well tested and established system of beliefs of constant of reality.

As to the group culture; this was a period of doubt and examination of all aspects of my life and in particular posed a great threat to my marriage (or so I thought at the time). I feel now without an underlying commitment and extreme tolerance on Jerry's part this period may have been very damaging. As it turned out it was just another development through suffering, reflection and negotiation. For a time I felt she did not understand the significance of what was happening to me and the whole of May 1987, although of course it was I that did not understand and I remember Jerry saying with astonishment at the time, 'How could I be so taken in and be fanatical?'.

I think my other close friends enjoyed my terror and found great interest and encouraged me in my impulsive conclusions and revelations about human behaviour and analysis of universal causes. All my friendships are still close ones and with time I have become a better listener and broader in my outlook, although no less committed and passionate, perhaps just more cautious and patient. (JX/C.82.S)

Interactions with clients brought this student face to face with his lived experience:

Working with clients has given first hand experience of how things can go wrong as well as right. Hopefully the former has not been too destructive on their part. The environment of training has been an excellent catalyst in developing interaction. Perhaps I would never have done so had I not changed direction and entered a 'people profession', to use a horrible expression. (JK/S.82.S)

Summary of subcategory 1d

A minority of students expressed the view that it was easy to be influenced by the nursing culture, which included the use of psychiatric nursing terminology relating to therapeutic intervention off the cuff in a patronizing way. A majority made the point that the training had influenced their interaction, level of social awareness and sensitivity to self and others, whereas a small section of the group, while accepting that they had improved their social skills, did not acknowledge any significant change in their lived experience.

A sizeable proportion made the point that the interaction within the group and during clinical placements had brought a change within their family situation as they started to be too analytical and critical of social situations, these resulting in family tensions at some stage during their training.

It is evident from their experiences that working with people at very close range influenced the students' perception of the world. This could add either richness or pain to their world. This created tension, which clearly affected their family life and circle of friends, in turn affecting the course, giving, for example, a need for clinical supervision.

Theory and practice: how do students bridge the gap?

This category has a bearing on the others as the sole purpose of training is the building of skills on existing knowledge that has been experienced and learned through sharing with others in different situations. It is directed towards personal experience and its relation to practice. The subcategories are:

- how students relate their experience to a plan of training, to arrive at a syllabus that is negotiable;
- the use of experiential learning to bridge the gap between theory and practice;
- the effects of client on the nurse's development;
- the importance of projects and lectures.

Subcategory 2a

The majority expressed the view that you cannot come out with a truly negotiable syllabus based on experience if you have not had the required experience or you are not aware of what is demanded. A skeletal framework is essential to build from:

> Experience of working with mentally ill people would help before starting your nurse training. In my own experience I had worked with people suffering from psychiatric problems which has helped me from the beginning of my chosen branch placement to feel a little more confident, as if I knew a little of what to experience. (BB/N.K2.S)
> I negotiated my training to include placements such as Rudolph Steiner School, the Child and Family Centre, Park View House (a centre for pregnant girls and teenage mothers). Seminars and private projects can all be centred around areas of personal interest but are self-directed, and in my view there was not enough tutor feedback on the content or ideas on other useful areas to investigate which might be

relevant to an individual's chosen topic. Feedback from the group, if led by a tutor knowledgeable in that field, was useful but depended heavily on the members of the group and their interest in the subject. (BB/N.K2.S)

It was not possible to negotiate the terms of the syllabus owing to the fact that the ENB guidelines, examination requirements and plan of training were already written. This view was shared by most of the students:

Because at the end of training we take an exam, it is important that we are directed towards certain goals. If allowed to negotiate the syllabus, then there has to be a way to negotiate how students are tested as well. (RM/N.82.S)

Placements we would have liked to have been to have not always been available, due to them not being approved by School or the ENB, such as certain social services facilities (like care and clusters, etc). We feel that if we had had a bit more guidance at the start rather than struggling to find what we needed to know, we would have had more time and energy to look outside the accepted institutional circuit. (BAC.LA.LO/C.82.S)

Negotiation was perceived as being possible through guidance, by looking at or questioning what was being done, step by step, and by looking retrospectively at what had been done. One group of 12 students made the point that negotiation is possible through reflection. Here are two of their comments:

My own personal experiences of a mental illness within the family lead me to become very interested in mental illness, therefore psychiatric nursing. The skills I acquired in dealing with this relative gave me insight into areas such as society's view of the mentally ill and the lack of good care given, (particularly within elderly). (BK/C.K2.S)

Having established a belief in the value of self-directed education I continued to participate in the process and was committed to ensuring I did my share of the work.

Looking back I can see how what I think is the strongest argument against self directed learning as described. This argument goes, 'In self directed learning, the students may not cover the areas that should be covered in preparation for qualification from student to professional practitioner.'

Our learner group, however, was given free choice in the early days of what we wished to cover in project work. Some of the topics covered were: grieving, suicide, schizophrenia, group/individual psychotherapy, physical abuse against women, homosexuality, behaviour therapy, alcoholism and a whole range more. The subjects covered were the very subjects the syllabus wanted covering, yet without looking at the syllabus these topics were covered in depth and with feeling. It seems that when a group of adults are self directing their education, their interest in this education keeps their mind tuned to what topics they should be looking at.

So this addressed how students can be on the right track. Any group however may not cover every area of the syllabus required. This is where the negotiation part of the process becomes important. It was very simple how this worked in our learner group. Towards the end of the first year in training it became obvious to the tutor that some important subjects had not been covered. This was brought to the attention of the group and a list of these subjects was then drawn up. By negotiation between the group members, all these subjects were covered. Later in the training in the final year, it became obvious that events in the world had dictated some new areas which should be covered if our course of training was to be comprehensive. These were then covered in a similar way.

So my experience shows that with the right people, people who respect the learners' ability as well as the tutors, a negotiation can take place which will lead to the covering of a comprehensive syllabus of education. (BUG./C.82.S)

A majority expressed the view that they would like to be informed about the requirements before negotiation. They wanted a kind of direction prior to negotiation:

It would help to see what we need to know, where we need to be and what level we need to work at by the time we qualify. This way we have a firm goal to work to and we can plan the work to achieve this. A vague set of rules and codes is no good to plan and work for. A level needs to be reached in both practice and theory and a firm goal set to be achieved. Although the assignment and continual assessment method decreases pressure, allowing for a more natural result, not enough pressure is exerted to check on levels of knowledge and skills, such as tests and exams (although I hate both of these I can see their value). (BT/N.K2.S)

For myself, I would have liked to have been given a copy of the ENB requirements for RMN training (i.e. amount of time needed to be spent on acute wards, elderly wards, rehab., etc), then to have been allowed to choose which wards to go on and which sequence to do them in!

> Not very realistic! Would give 'allocations' a few headaches! Plan – identify certain 'core' requirements for RMN training – obviously, everybody will need a certain minimum amount of experience in different clinical areas, such as elderly, acute, etc. (CK/C.82.S)

Exposing the planning team to the students would hopefully make a change towards a kind of negotiation. This was the view of one student:

> I feel the course has been flexible in meeting my needs as a student. By introducing students to the team of people responsible in structuring the syllabus, perhaps the syllabus could become increasingly negotiable. However in my experience and as a year representative, the majority of students are quite passive and apathetic when it comes to any extra involvement necessary to the course. (HT/C.K2.S)

Negotiation would leave the plan to subjective experience, which was expressed by this one student:

> The experience gained by the students in their life before coming into nurse training may be seen as useful but not necessarily as a means of negotiating a plan of training.
>
> Unless one has had direct experience with the area of work in which one is specializing (either as an employee or as a member of the public, recipient), then life experience becomes a very subjective and individual concern. What we are actually referring to is 'personal' life experience, which is often subject to individual values and interpretations that may have been constructed from negative as well as positive life experience.
>
> The application of life experience to the clinical plan of training, which is often more likely to be subject to utilitarian considerations, where individual values, prejudice and judgements are rejected or challenged and thereby neutralized. (MD/N.K2.S)

Summary of subcategory 2a

The feeling expressed by a majority was that they needed to have had the required experience and awareness of what was demanded from the course before any meaningful negotiation could take place. A large number of students made the point that the syllabus was not conducive to negotiation as the rules for examinations, the control of clinical experiences and the training plan were under the direction of the ENB. A large group made the point that, looking at the training retrospectively, there was a kind of negotiation, some expressing the view that negotiation was possible when a step-by-step approach was taken. The view that negotiation would have been possible if the planning team were exposed to the student group was made by a minority. One student observed that negotiation would leave planning a 'subjective' and simply personal experience.

This section raised the following issues:

1. How can students negotiate if they do not know what is demanded of them?
2. There is a need to know the ENB guidelines and the course require-ment before planning can take place.

Subcategory 2b

These two students expressed the view that reality is on the ward – theory and School cannot ever prepare them:

> I don't think anything really from School can quite prepare you for when you first get onto a ward and encounter that reality. What I feel I did gain from this though was being more aware of how others see you and interpret your verbal and non-verbal communication. This I feel can be taken with you into practice. (BB/C.82.S)
>
> The use of experiential learning does not necessarily bridge the gap between theory and practice, for a number of possible reasons. The nature of theory is that it often seeks to explain human experience in overtly scientific, and sociological language, which in practical common sense understanding bears no relationship to experience in everyday life as perceived by lay persons and professionals alike. (MDK./N.82.S)

With skilful facilitation and with a group willing to participate, the gap can, however, be bridged. This idea was shared by a minority of students:

> Yes, provided the links are clearly explained, i.e. reasoning behind an exercise and considerable time for evaluation after it (plus a skilled facil-itator). Certain experiential exercises, particularly role play, I found frightening to contemplate in a group of 13 and have avoided it. I feel the choice of experiential learning styles and the timing of them has to be right or their value can be limited. (RE/S.82.S)
>
> Experiential learning should bridge the gap between theory and practice as examples of the application of theory in practice are shared within the group and techniques and skills are acquired by all. Debate, role play, project presentation are all effective ways of achieving this

and need to be done much more than in present training. Direction still needs to be provided from tutors, and tutors' experience in nursing (if they haven't forgotten it all) is equally if not more important and must be shared to provide an understanding of what is important. (BK/D.82.S)

The practical situations on the ward helped to clarify the theory. The view was shared by these two students:

Experiential learning has been my main method of learning. Ward experience has given me a foundation on which to build the 'theory'. (KX/N.82.S)

I think that experiential learning can bridge the gap between theory and practice if you have good clinical experiences and mentors. Whilst in the community with a CPN, he was very well read and had researched different approaches and theories of psychiatric nursing and used them with his interactions with patients. To see him work and then discuss the approaches and what information he would get from the client was very informative and made me realize the information and experience required to deal with some patients and their problems. (BK/N.K2.S)

This encouraged reflection, questioned the nurse's belief system and created a feeling of empathy. These are the embodiment of a skilled practitioner, a view shared by 12 of the students. Here are two examples:

An experience which can be shared by either a group member or an invited speaker can only serve to increase the learner's awareness of that topic above what it would be if the information were presented in a purely theoretical manner.

Experiential learning is the process of learning, stated Bugental; we recognize that a good knowledge base can only increase the effectiveness of a practitioner but we then address how this knowledge must be used. He states that only when knowledge is incorporated into the everyday skills of a practitioner can this knowledge be used by the humanistic therapist to the benefit of this client. The knowledge must become part of the person's skills – part of the person. Only through experiential learning can this process be achieved. (UG/C.82.S)

At times at the beginning of the course, the content which was discussed, people's personal experiences, worries, past experience, seemed to be discussed openly and freely as though a lid was released and letting out repressed feelings, thoughts, etc. I felt uncomfortable in this situation, a group of strangers who seemed to be pouring their hearts out to one another; one almost felt guilty as though one was expected to dig deep into past experience and divulge one's own secrets.

Often I would leave School, head buzzing with what had gone on previously, trying to make sense of it, more often than not successful, and there began a dread of not wanting to go into School so as not to face the confusion of not knowing how to make sense of it.

Once on the ward it seemed to slot in what had previously gone on in School, faced with people pouring out their problems, talking about wanting to end their life, and drawing on what happened within the classroom I was able to draw on that experience and handle the situation which previously I would have had no idea and be detrimental to the situation. (HO/C.82.S)

Experiential learning can thus bridge the gap, but students do not have enough practical experience to draw on. The lecturers should work partly on the ward to know the problem. This view was aired by these two students:

Experiential learning is very important to make sense of some of the theory but we don't have enough practical experience to draw on. I think the course would be more effective reversed, more practical than theory; a day release system maybe with a few study blocks a year would be much more beneficial.

There is still a very big gap between practice and theory; some of it cannot be bridged because it just isn't used in practice (so is there really much point in spending so much time on these subjects?). I also think that it may be more beneficial for lecturers and students if the lecturers worked partly on wards so that they can more appreciate the gap we face. (SG/N.82.S)

I feel that experiential learning can bridge the gap between theory and practice although often being a student, experiential learning is not always offered. More often than not the student is only of observational capacity. Experiential learning needs to be an ongoing trait throughout training rather than being made available in the last year, as it is now. It is an important link between theory and practice, allowing one to know the facts, but also be part of the practical (realistic) side. (MK/D.82.S)

It became evident after training that this was a difficult bridge to create, a view shared thus by one student:

> Experiential learning can form a bridge but it is my experience that this bridge is very difficult to create and the process is a great deal slower than I expected. It is only in the final six months of training and after registration that the theory/practice gap begins to truly close. Much of this is due I feel to the removal of some of the student cushioning and the uptake of responsibility. I do not feel this to be detrimental but an important phase of consolidation. (HT/S.82.S)

Summary of subcategory 2b

A minority of students made the point that the reality could only be encountered on the ward, School activity could not bridge the gap, and that personal experience could be too subjective to apply to clinical situations. A large proportion, viewing from a different angle, saw the ward as the source of experience that could be used for explaining situations and for clarifying what had been covered in theoretical sessions.

They also stressed that they did not have enough practical experience to draw from and that lecturers should be partly involved in the clinical environment in order to understand their situation. A large proportion stated that experiential learning, if effectively facilitated, would encourage reflection, help to question belief systems and create a feeling of empathic understanding; these are the embodiment of a skilled practitioner. The issues raised were:

1. Personal experiences could be too subjective to apply to clinical situations.
2. Ward situations could help to clarify theories taught in School.
3. Lecturers needed to work alongside students in clinical situations.

Subcategory 2c

The interaction with clients helped to create insight and feelings of empathic understanding. The situation could then have a knock-on effect on the confidence and mood of the students, creating a feeling of negation and cynicism, a view expressed by these two students:

> Working with clients has given me a lot of insight, the opportunity to be empathic. I do however often feel overwhelmed by distress which has a knock-on effect on my own mood and confidence. It is very easy to be negative on the ward. (TX/D.82.S)
>
> Every day's interaction, whether with clients, fellow staff members or whoever, have an effect on one's development. I suppose, especially whilst working on acute ward, I became more cynical of some clients

which before I was accepting of people's illnesses, not questioning any motives, but especially after spending time on acute wards after discussion following projects, 'sick role' and personal responsibility, it threw another light on the situation – do people take upon the sick role to escape responsibility, etc.? Even though I have said I have become more accepting, I suppose I look deeper than previously into all aspects of the client which may provoke/cause mental illness – family, social environment. (WK/C.82.S)

The experience could influence the nurses' belief systems, in that it helped them to accommodate others, as reported by two students:

I found it very difficult working with battered women as it brought into question my own beliefs. I became very frustrated with what I experienced and while my beliefs did not change fully, I have had to widen them in order to take into account my experience. (FC/N.82.S)

I have problems coming to terms with the expected situation where the nurse 'detaches themself from the client emotionally'. It is my belief that to ignore any aspect of the self will lead to incongruence which can have a negative effect on the therapeutic relationship. It is my belief that every interaction has an effect on me, be it either a reinforcement of already held beliefs or a challenging of those beliefs that need dealing with. (UG/C.82.S)

The interventions with clients could help in the students' personal development and assist in the forming of relationships with others. These interactions also helped in putting the students in touch with their own feelings and assisted them in coping with the ups and downs of life events. These ideas were expressed by a majority of students, these being two quotes:

It has also helped me to see things from the other person's side and it has helped me to reflect on my own life and experiences. In some cases I have realized that some things I did, I did them and learn from these mistakes. (CW/N.K2.S)

I feel probably the experience gained from clients is to a great extent a reflection of my own ability to cope, sustain my own health and be able to be with others and relate to others in a meaningful way; then the effects are as varied as the clients I have known. Each meeting adds to my knowledge of human behaviour/feelings and broadly speaking the human condition, giving me more ways of understanding/formulating my picture of the human world and my place in it, as well as my increased awareness of my own psychic noise or making more sense/different sense of the ripples of my own past experience. To restore internal conflicts is not a process of smoothing out the past's ups and downs: it is more importantly preparation for the ups and downs of the future.

To list the effects would be pointless, to acknowledge them is enough. (JX/C.82.S)

Good and bad experience with clients have fortified my armour. The range and variety of people I have encountered have allowed me to move beyond a certain boundary of views, thus expanding my experience and awareness. Cross-cultural experience has occurred in a way which I might never have experienced. I have been 'taken for a ride' and in a sense abused, which has also helped. I have also had unlimited good experiences adding to my motivation and compassion. (KJ/C.82.S)

Working with clients influenced the development of skills and created an awareness of one's own limitations, as the majority of students described:

Clients I have had quite close working relationships with I have found I have learned a lot from, about the awareness of my skills and limitations. Sometimes this can be quite negative; if you feel you weren't that good in a situation, you can feel quite deskilled, but this would be a positive thing because may be you did lack skills in that situation. It's just that after a 'bad' experience sometimes you feel you just lack skills, full stop. I have found though that through experience has come knowledge, which can be applied in subsequent situations. (BG/C.82.S)

Clients do have an effect on both my personal and professional development through:

i)   gained confidence and skillls in therapeutic interaction
ii) comments received from clients.

Clients enable me to look at myself in more depth and be aware of individuality and the need for a non-judgmental approach. Has taught me how to interact with people from all walks of life, both professionally and personally. (BW/D.82.S)

One comments described how the students had been helped to see clients as individuals:

The most profound impact which client interaction has had on my own experience is that those suffering from mental illness are not a homogeneous group of people who experience a universal pathological phenomena and who all present and express the same 'symptomatology' on admission. (MD/N.K2.S)

Summary of subcategory 2c

A small proportion of students felt that the clients could create in them a feeling of cynicism and that this could result in a negative view of themselves and others. In some cases, they had to accommodate others within their own beliefs system regardless of their personal values.

A great majority of students expressed the view that their interventions with clients helped in their personal development, assisted them in coping with their own situations and put them in touch with their own feelings, thus creating social awareness. The contact with others, albeit painful, enriched their lived experiences.

A large proportion stated that clients influenced the development of their own skills in caring and made them aware of their limitations. One student made the point that the interactions had made him see clients as individuals and not as a generic group of illnesses.

As expected in this kind of learning situation, the points made are that:

1. Skills are learnt through interaction with patients.
2. Clinical situations also assist in personal development.

Subcategory 2d

Lectures suited a minority. They enjoyed listening and thinking, covering the groundwork:

> As previously stated I seem to have a problem with project work. There is a natural revulsion to written work! I have a feeling that written work is vanity. This stems purely from my faith. Life's purpose is not to pass on whims and ideas but to discover the unchanging truth through living not intellectualization. Lectures probably suit me better. I enjoy hearing ideas and views in a discussion setting rather than reading endless viewpoints. (RK/C.82.S)
>
> Help to make you think and develop in areas not normally explored. They also help you to expand your way of thinking and provide a greater knowledge base. (NON./C.K2.S)

A large proportion found it difficult to learn from lectures as it depended on the lecturers and the type of information given:

> On the whole I do not feel I have learnt a lot from lectures; they have mainly pointed me in the right direction and given references for subjects. (CW/N.K2.S)

> Projects can be useful to reinforce information. Lectures have been quite disappointing during our course as often lecturers haven't turned up, etc. (WW/N.K2.S)

Projects could be challenging, helping in the development of research skills and in obtaining in-depth information. The presentation could be difficult but it developed the student's confidence within the group. Such views were expressed by a large proportion of the students:

> The first few projects were pure hell, having not written anything to compare with a project for 10 years.
> The research was enjoyable; collecting information together, interviewing people and setting the interviews up was all a new experience. I felt awkward about this, but it built up confidence and I was able to ask of others – time, questions, something which I have always found difficult.
> The presentation of projects were of a high standard and politely received by fellow members, making polite comments and positive criticism. It was a shame that we had to cram them into such a short space of time: it was hardgoing for those listening as well as those presenting the projects.
> Lectures were again valuable experiences; not so much sociology, which we covered in the classroom amongst members of the group. Invited people who came in and gave personal accounts of their culture, religion and beliefs were beneficial and gave you space to question your own prejudices and beliefs. (WJ/C.82.S)
> Don't like doing presentations but feel that they do help you to become more confident and conversant. (BK/N.K2.S)
> Project work has helped me develop my knowledge and understanding of a lot of things and pushed me academically. (SD/N.K2.S)

Projects tended to be a hindrance, unmotivated and not satisfying, the view shared by these two students:

> I tend to regard projects as a hindrance rather than as a positive learning opportunity. I think that in a purely academic qualification, project work as a requirement of the course would make more sense. In this training you are assessed on your clinical work reports, assessments. The clinical placements take up much of the training but you are also expected to undertake a fair degree of academic work. I feel sometimes that some of the tutors' reasoning for project work, e.g. teaching experience, sharing knowledge with the group, is a mask for

actually checking that people are putting in the required academic input. (ED/C.82.S)

Projects are OK when they have a purpose – often it just seems to be jumping through hoops. So I get disinterested, unmotivated and do the minimum to get by and feel dissatisfied with myself because of it. When they have a point and genuinely got airmed at educating yourself and the group, they are really worthwhile and you feel a sense of responsibility to do something properly. (NOM/D.82.S)

Summary of subcategory 2d

A proportion of the students expressed the view that they enjoyed listening to lectures, these being found to be a useful tool when covering new ground. The point that lectures were difficult to learn from was also made by a large number of respondents.

Doing projects could be seen as challenging and helpful in the development of research skills, as well as giving the students an in-depth information of the subject area.

The presentation of projects was seen as very demanding, but this helped to build the confidence of the student. Information and knowledge gathered from projects could help the students to explain some clinical situations. A small proportion found project work to be a hindrance and not satisfying.

The issues raised were:

1. Lectures and projects could be useful tools, lectures being good for imparting information.
2. Projects helped to develop study skills and in-depth knowledge, and the presentation of projects helped to build the students' level of confidence.

The role of mentorship/supervision: how do students learn within this mode? This question targets the perceptions of self and other during the 3-year course. The subcategories were:

- evaluation by peers and others;
- mentorship and supervision;
- role and identity during training.

Subcategory 3a

Opinion on the helpfulness of group members was divided, an equal number reporting positive and negative feedback. Some saw peer comments as constructive, supportive and the yardstick by which to measure performance:

> The feedback/evaluation of peers has been a yardstick from which I have measured my performance or ability and development. The feedback from others, i.e. qualified staff, has been, depending on my trust of that person, a way of monitoring my skill acquisition and creative adaptability.
>
> It is an important tool and much-needed encouragement when offered with respect and care. If it is not given in such a way, I have distanced myself from it or indicated the source of usually a personalized dumping of the others' emotional distractions. (JX/C.82.S)
>
> I have always felt that I have had a good evaluation from my peers, who have passed on encouragement, criticism and different ways to look and do things. (BB/N.K2.S)

Others, however, were not as impressed:

> A bit false really. Who is going to say, in front of everyone, so and so is a dick-head? (BM/T.K2.S)
>
> Most of the evaluation and feedback given to me has been to emphasize the positive aspects and attributes I've shown and not pointed out things which I may have been doing wrong. Instead of telling someone they need to work, they just gossip about it behind your back but not help you overcome these. (BG/C.82.S)

There is some evidence that the students themselves became able to see the peer group in more objectives terms as the course developed:

> I think people have divorced themselves from the initial artificiality of the group as being some mystical, all-important sacred magic circle. This was a false concept that led us down a path of frustration and inadequacy. We have grown apart, thank God! Things are more geared to personal development and everyone's got their eye on the future. Everyone's got more 'real' and less 'what shall we do today?' We have taken more control. (ZX/D.82.S)
>
> I think that at the end of this training you tend to be less judgmental than at the start of the course. Old stereotypes die hard! (MD/T.K2.S)

Only one student expressed the view that she had experienced hostility:

From the beginning of the Project 2000 course, students have had to battle with negative and resentful comments from nurses and various other disciplines on the wards. In this climate it has been difficult to function, and Project 2000 nurses have felt a need to prove themselves. It is difficult to judge just how beneficial theoretical knowledge will be at the expense of practical knowledge at this stage, I would say the time for evaluation will be when we begin as staff nurses. At this particular moment in time I would say we are ill prepared for staff nurse responsibilities without the backup of a mentor or some other form of support. (NON/N.K2.S)

Summary of subcategory 3a

Of the 86 students who commented on this issue, opinion was clearly divided, an equal number believing in the usefulness of peer feedback and its lack of honesty. There is some indication of a greater awareness of the nature of group influence as the course developed, and only one student reported experiencing hostile comments. The quality of feedback, in terms of its honesty and openness, appears to be the main issue.

Subcategory 3b

The majority of students saw the supervisions as being supportive, respectful and enabling. For supervision to work, the students' commitment is needed:

I think I've learnt a lot about supervising from my supervisors. On the whole my supervisors have been excellent. But other times they were more interested in their images as a supervisors; for example, they filled in reports for their benefit, not for mine. I've found the most successful supervisors are the ones who are willing to encourage what I think are assets and help me to work on my deficiencies. Having been a 'mentor' myself I've found the commitment of the person being 'mentored' important. So perhaps the areas where I've found my supervisors lacking is where I haven't been committed. (GK/C.82.S)

I feel that this placement has been an invaluable experience for me. Due to taking my finals early I was in a position to use this experience to the full, look at my strengths and weaknesses and work on these whilst working within a team of nurses that worked independently.

Supervision was excellent, having sessions every few weeks with my supervisor. However, informal supervision was available and used all the time by myself with my supervisor, mentor and other members of staff.

Caseload. I keyworked half a dozen clients – the majority of which I followed through from admission to discharge. Working within the multi-disciplinary team I was treated as a permanent member of staff but I always had the support and supervision of staff if needed. The opportunities for assessment/admission/sectioning and the decisions that come with them were more than plenty with quite a quick turnover of clients.

Management exercise. On such a ward it is not possible to be the shift manager on your own due to the interdependence of staff, which I feel is very positive. Thus when problems arise on the ward you are not on your own.

Mentoring. I mentored two Common Foundation Programme students, each for a 4 week period – conducting supervision on a weekly basis, filling the forms in and arranging appropriate visits to other areas in the mental health service. (HW/D.82.S)

Clinical supervisions were good, but the contact with the link teacher was minimal to the point of non-existence. During supervision, the personality of the clinical supervisors played a great part. They made the students aware of clinical opportunities for practice. This view was expressed by clearly two-thirds of the students who took part, for example:

This is very important to ensure safety on the wards and to enable students to expand their academic and practical knowledge on and off the ward and using their supervisors as sounding boards for new ideas. Supervision from School is also important to keep a link for the 3 months' placements. I'm afraid after the middle of the 2nd year this has been denied me as I've not had a visit from any tutor while on the wards. Do they only turn up when there are problems? (FK/N.82.S)

It is my experience that a good mentor, i.e. a nurse who understands that the role of a mentor is to help students gain as much from their placements as possible, is by: a) being made aware of every opportunity which arises to either practise new skills or improve on skills already acquired, b) giving guidance on policies and procedures to enable students to put theory into practice, c) personality is an important issue. If there happens to be a clash of personalities then a whole placement can be wasted. This has been addressed in some areas: you choose your own mentor (a person with whom you feel you can develop a rapport). Some mentors have been particularly aware of their responsibilities and have held teaching sessions for their students. It does not surprise me, in the light of the inconsistency between mentors, that a Project 2000 nurse can qualify without every having given an injection; from my experience it could quite easily happen. (BW/N.K2.S)

One of the students made the point that it would ideally be preferable to have the same supervisor for the 3 years, making it the extended role of the personal tutor:

Essential for personal growth. Ideally I would have liked a facility for weekly/fortnightly supervision in School – would have liked formal supervision from the same person on a regular basis, from beginning to end of training. In this way would have had more continuity on a personal level. Extended version of personal tutor! Supervision on wards from clinical staff can be good but there is no continuity in terms of assessing personal progress and often it is more helpful to talk to someone outside that clinical area. Problems: (1) do nurse tutors have the skills to perform such a role?, (2) do they have the time? (MW/C.82.S)

A small minority believed that the role of supervisor was overrated; they preferred to approach the nearest qualified staff available. This was the view of these three students:

On only one ward have I needed to rely on my supervisor for support and supervision whilst I have been on a ward. Everywhere else I have been able to rely on whichever qualified staff were on at the time, to ensure I got the most from each learning experience on the ward. I have found the latter far more beneficial, partly because of the immediacy of the event makes it easier to assimilate the different issues involved, and rarely because the supervisor's spontaneity and creativity, as well as my own, lend to a better learning experience. (UG/C.82.S)

I have never had a mentor or even felt the need for one. Supervision I have usually found good but I prefer feedback from the ward staff in general rather than one individual. Often when looking for advice or guidance I go to the first person at hand rather than seek out my supervisor, so the importance of their role diminishes. As a general rule I think the more confident you are on a ward and the more able you are to communicate with staff, the less important a supervisor is. (BK/D.82.S)

One student reported a difficulty arising from the supervisor's personality. Supervision had been cancelled because of the supervisor's lack of commitment and level of stress. The student's performance could thus be hampered by the knowledge and insight of the supervisor. This might further be affected by personal feeling:

One of the difficulties I have had with my supervisor is that she is constantly stressed, very busy and very assertive. I find it hard to be assertive with her, to ask for support and time. Our weekly hourly supervision times seem to be constantly reduced or cancelled due to other commitments. I feel that I have to be more aware of her needs rather than mine, and because I have a natural tendency to put others' needs before my own, I find it difficult to assert my own. However, I feel that during the allocation I have become increasingly assertive, along with my increasing confidence. (WL/D.82.S)

One student would like to take part in selecting the supervisor for personality reasons:

To be there if needed. Very important. But the practice of the mentor and supervisor being selected before you reach the ward seems silly. You need to know that you can form some kind of relationship (i.e. trust, confidence – just a 'professional' friendship) with the mentor/supervisor. Only you and he can know that, not the ward manager. (CL/C.82.S)

Supervision could be perceived as a hindrance and as meeting the need of the supervisor:

This depends on the ward; I've had mentors that are not very supportive but have been given a student because they are in the process of completing their 998 course (Teaching & Assessing Course). It's easier to complete the course if they have a student. (LW/N.K2.S)

Still really not clear where mentor differs from supervisor and I don't think I've been allocated a mentor during the course. The effectiveness of supervision seems to depend on how well you relate together as individuals, on the attitude of the supervisor to the task of supervising students (at worst some seem to see it as a hindrance and are eager to get the business done, e.g. reports and send you on your way). Clinically, supervision often seems to be given by a number of staff, and depending on whom you are working with that shift seems to work adequately. It is helpful to feel you can approach someone when needing support. Sometimes this has been my supervisor and sometimes not. (ED/C.82.S)

Summary of subcategory 3b

A large proportion of students valued their clinical supervision in that it assisted them to link theory and practice through a reflection on clinical cases. The commitment of the students was seen as essential for the supervision to be meaningful. The supervisor's personality was held to a major factor in the relationship; students made the point that they wished to take part in the selection of their supervisor rather than the selection being made by the clinical manager. One student said that it would be preferable to have the same supervisor for the 3 years' training, making this the extended role of the personal tutor.

A great number of students made the point that link teachers to clinical areas had minimal input and that they would like their assistance in clinical settings.

Three of the students stated that the role of the supervisor was overrated. They preferred to approach any qualified staff who were on duty at that time rather than having a specified individual to deal with clinical issues.

Some students also made the point that supervision sessions were sometimes cancelled because the supervisor was too stressed and that they were hampered by the knowledge and skills of the supervisors. In some cases, supervision was perceived to be a hindrance.

The issues raised were:

1. the role of the supervisor and the link teacher in relation to clinical practice – the theory–practice link;
2. students' commitment to supervision;
3. whether having a specified supervisor was a hindrance;
4. whether students should have the same clinical supervisor for the whole course.

Subcategory 3c

Not surprisingly, a large proportion of the students' feeling of confidence depended on the clinical situations in which they were involved and on how much of a contribution they made. Responses to this question highlighted the problems attached to learning a new and often demanding role while also working. Some students drew attention to role conflicts, pointing out different expectations as well as the conflict between being trusted as a team member and being 'watched' as a student:

> There is a sense in which you, as a student, are both a member of a staff team on a ward as well as an outsider – in that one's time is limited, one has a prescribed area of legal responsibilities different from other staff, and one is under the dual judicial of School and hospital management. So the role often envisaged for you by staff on the ward

is that you are a trainee staff nurse and should as far as possible be immersed in a staff nurse's activities with supervision.

The identity, the internal construct of the students regarding their role may be very different and they may feel themselves forced into a conflict, where the role envisaged for them by the staff team is unacceptable, possibly due to practices which they find questionable. Taking on fully the staff construct of role can involve the student in feelings of loosened identity or compromised identity. Similarly the conflict which can emerge between staff and student where discrepancies regarding role are present can raise stress levels. So the conflict can be internal (with outward conformity) or external (with disagreements in the open). I have also had the experience of finding myself in broad agreement with ward philosophy and staff attitudes, but finding it difficult to identify myself with a role in the ward environment, particularly where one can see qualified staff unable to fulfil roles, this visibility being due to underresourcing. (RD/D.82.S)

The role and identity of the student nurse is somewhat confused. In some clinical areas the student nurse is seen as a professional who has certain capabilities and can work with supervision in a self directed way. In other areas the student nurse is seen as someone who needs 'watching'. This makes an identified role difficult to find. I've found that it takes time to find a compromise between what I want to do and what I think I need and what the ward and the staff will allow me to do. As an identity of a student nurse it again depends on the setting and environment, which may be socially or in the educational establishment or in the clinical environment. (GK/C.82.S)

The lack of knowledge about clinical situations affected the students' level of confidence. This depended on the level of their contribution, which might in turn be influenced by the level of morale on the ward:

I sometimes feel very insignificant and at other times quite important and valued. I think perhaps that this is due to knowledge in certain circumstances, whether you have any or not pertaining to a particular situation and in relation to this the contribution you can make in that same situation, affecting your feeling of self worth and confidence. (THG/D.82.S)

Feel that as my training has progressed I have lost confidence in myself. Partly due to low morale and changes taking place within nursing in general, Project 2000, community moves, etc. My 'role' as a student nurse seems to have differed, depending on which ward/clinical area I have worked in; i.e. my role has tended to reflect the attitudes of qualified staff I have worked with. (BW/C.82.S)

Identity changed according to situation, the student displaying what was expected at that time. A large section of students extended their role to suit the situation, of which the following are examples:

I know on wards I try to play the expected role to make life easier for myself, but I don't feel this poses a threat to my identity. So far I have found it possible to maintain my identity and make some impression, though not always well liked as an individual, while changing roles to some extent to suit the ward and School environment. (BK/D.82.S)

During training we take on the role of student and to a lesser extent our identify alters. I myself have noticed a change throughout training in the area of my identity in that I have developed the identity of being a nurse instead of playing at being a nurse. (NON/T.K2.S)

Three students reported that the constant change of allocation made it difficult to settle and to establish their identity; for example:

Roles have been fixed. However identity is continually changing, I think due to levels of stress from never being able to stay somewhere long enough to find yourself, your place, your role or your friends. (CW/N.K2.S)

To the following students, identity was seen as being developmental, and what they put in during training changed with experience:

I consider that my role during training has changed as I've gone along. For the first ward or two I felt I was there more as an observer than anything else, but as I've progressed it's become apparent that as a student I have an opinion worth listening to, that I have a role as a member of staff on the ward, actually being a nurse, a counsellor, an advocate, whatever. Not only has my perception of my role changed but others' perceptions also, to the point of other staff saying, 'well you are a third year now' for example. Again, though, a lot of this depends on the staff you are working with.

However as time has gone on, especially after you have worked on a ward for a while, you do get an identity as a member of staff on that ward, no matter how temporary you are, an identity given to you by both staff and clients. Usually this identity is limited to the confines of being 'a student', which can be quite comforting, but on the other hand it can be frustrating. On one occasion I have actually felt an independent part of a team with similar responsibilities and workloads of permanent staff, which was a gradual process and hence nonthreatening. This was the most beneficial experience in my training and went hand in hand with a lot of support and supervision. This was on [Ward X] when it served as an in-patient facility. (OK/C.82.S)

No problems with roles and identity during training and as clinical/theoretical/practical experience grows so does your confidence and ability to work using your own initiative whatever your expectations are. You only get out of a course what you are prepared to put in. (DM/T.K2.S)

Being assertive could help one to retain one's identify throughout training, a view shared by a minority of students:

My role and identify has remained reasonably static throughout my training. I was reasonably self-aware before I commenced training. I have found it easier to interact with others since training and can now put up with idiots at parties easier than before. (SK/N.82.S)

I very rarely felt like a 'student nurse', feeling rather an individual with certain expectations. Those expectations can be changed by assertion of self and understanding your environment, always respectful of others' experience, from that of staff feeling all student nurses like gossip and incestuous social lives to that of being a committed responsible adult.

As to my own identity, I felt 'I can't wait to qualify'; my feeling is neither that of a student nor that of a nurse. Before I had a social identity; now I am in some no-man's land. (JX/C.82.S)

The following three students perceived the role as student as being good to hide behind. Being used as a pair of hands, as well as the supernumerary status of the student, was seen as detrimental to an individual's experience. These were the views shared by these three students:

It is easy to hide behind the role of students, to hide from doing things we don't want to or situations that we are unsure of. Conventional students are often seen as a 'pair of hands', particularly on elderly wards, and this can often become drudgery rather than a learning experience in the best sense of the word. (BX/N.82.S)

I think often we are seen as pairs of hands first and students second, particularly in the first half of training. I feel as a student that I have a lesser status than other staff but I feel being a mature student helps me to identify more with a lot of clients. (KM/C.82.S)

Supernumerary status has presented some problems in clinical areas, with confusion over what students can and cannot do. In certain areas this has been detrimental to students, who are deprived of learning opportunities because of alack of clear instructions as to their supernumerary role. (MD/N.K2.S)

Summary of subcategory 3c

A large group of students expressed the view that their identity depended on the clinical situation. If they knew what they were doing, this enhanced their confidence, the contribution they were making influencing their perception of self. In some cases, it was best to be a silent participant in order not to be put down.

Identity and role changed according to the clinical situation and what was expected of them, stated a large group of students. A good proportion experienced a feeling of conflict in that what was expected from them was not how they felt within themselves. A constant change of clinical situation and allocation affected a large proportion of the students. They made the point that it was difficult to establish oneself in a short space of time. A minority perceived self-identity as being developmental and a function of how they participated during their training.

A small group of students felt that being assertive helped them to retain their identity during training. A minority perceived the role of student as being a good thing to hide behind; they were used as a pair of hands on the clinical areas, but this supernumerary status had been detrimental to their clinical experience.

An important issue raised was whether clinical allocations should be longer to allow students to develop their clinical skills and confidence. What was expected by the School from students needed to be clearly stated to the clinical staff.

Learning in the clinical setting: how the students relate to the real-life learning environment

This category consists of the following subcategories:

- the position of the student nurse in relation to other professionals, as perceived by the student;
- whether self-direction was too demanding;
- allocation and relationships with others in the clinical setting.

These factors influenced the development of students during clinical placements.

Subcategory 4a

These student nurses perceived themselves to be of low social status in comparison with other health workers. They viewed this as a reflection upon them of how the other nursing staff were valued by other care workers. Because of these observations, a large proportion of the students felt that their views about clients were not considered to be valid in the making of clinical decisions. Here are two examples:

> As a student you 'command' a low position in the ward hierarchy. This can change with time as trust builds up. It can often rest on the type of professional you are dealing with and if they are prepared to impart bits of their knowledge or keep it to themselves. Professionals can often close ranks on you as a student and you can have little effect of this process. (GK/N.82.S)
>
> On the whole the position of the student nurse appears to be seen as someone who gets in the way and often as an extra support worker. However, I have on the whole had good placements during which staff and other professionals have recognized my learning needs and treated me as a member of the multi-disciplinary team. However, I believe students are better treated and respected in mental health in comparison to general nursing. (CW/N.K2.S)

The treatment of student nurses depended upon the ward to which they were allocated. Their contributions were valued, although they might be considered in some cases as a threat to qualified staff as a result of their ideas being more up to date. This observation was reported by a fair proportion of the students:

> I have found the position of the student nurse in relation to other professionals differs from ward to ward. You are either listened to and treated much the same as the permanent staff by medics: whether they take what you say and do something with it or they choose to ignore it and treat you as just 'nurses'.
>
> Some wards value student contribution, others treat you as a pair of hands usually depending on the hierarchical structure and the opinions of the ward manager. He may feel threatened by students, especially those willing to put forward new ideas or whose theoretical and research knowledge is more up to date; he will then under threat cling to past experience and knowledge, disregarding anything the students may put forward (or permanent staff). (EW/C.82.S)
>
> Depends upon which ward or allocation one goes on. Personally on most of my allocations I have been regarded as an individual and made

to feel a member of the team, although limitations as a student are always made clear. On other placements expectations are high, with comments such as 'students should bring along new ideas', yet on other wards student knowledge is put down: 'you are not expected to know as you are only a student'. Often difficult to get a balance, wanting to get involved (experiential learning) yet having to be aware of role of student. (AL/D.82.S)

From their observations, they felt that they were respected and accepted as valued members of the team during the third year of training. This was the basic observation of a great number of the students:

It depends which ward or environment you work in and how far into your training you are. I feel that as a third year and part of rostered service I have been accepted more as part of the team and my opinion has counted and you are not treated as the errand girl, as you probably were on occasions throughout the first two years. However you are always aware that you are the student and have to perform to reach certain goals to achieve objectives in your blue booklet. Also the fact that we flit around so much makes you feel as though you don't belong anywhere. (WS/N.K2.S)

The student nurse appears to me to be one of the least respected groups of 'professionals' for the first two years, and then in the third year you are given more respect whether or not it is earned. The student nurse with 18 months' experience is given less respect than the nursing assistant with 3 days experience. There seem to be stereotype student nurses who don't really know their rear end from their elbow, and sometimes you have to fight against this stereotype before you gain any respect. (GK/C.82.S)

This depends on the ward and the attitude of the 'other professionals'. Some look upon you as basically not worth bothering with; others appear to value your opinions and your actions. This gets better, generally, the farther you get into your training. I feel that the role of a student is important to maintain awareness of permanent staff of different attitudes, approaches and viewpoints. (DS/S.82.S)

This one student expressed the opinion that being limited in knowledge and lacking in experience did not stop her being respected by the team:

I have always felt well respected as a student nurse, to have had a role in the multidisciplinary team. Socially I have felt inadequate and also very much aware of the limitations of my knowledge and experience. I have felt that professionals enjoy conveying their knowledge to students and being questioned. (AG/D.82.S)

The observations made by a large proportion of the groups was that knowing the basic skills made them credible in clinical situations. Knowing basic skills helped to build their confidence:

> In order to gain credibility, students need to be proficient in the basic skills of psychiatric nurses; without these skills their opinions are not valued. Nurses will not be confident enough either even if they possess the theoretical knowledge to be assertive and push their own views forward. Confidence comes from knowing the basics and being valued by other professionals. (BM/N.K2.S)
>
> If one thinks about what one is saying and has the knowledge to back it up, I think the student nurse is treated as a respected member of the nursing profession. They have to take into account political ward environment, not be too idealistic though strive towards it; it is not always possible to achieve and one should accept this. (WL/C.82.S)

A small proportion pointed out that students could create their own position amongst other health professionals. This depended on how they projected themselves in clinical situations:

> The position of the student nurse in comparison with other profes-sionals depended largely on where I was working at the time and ranged from prodigal son to an awkward child, the second of which is how I felt with the School of Nursing.
>
> I also believe that the students themselves can create their own social position in relation to other professionals, depending on how they project or assert themselves. This is their own responsibility. I cannot think of a clinical placement where I did not feel of value. (JX/C.82.S)
>
> This varies dependent upon the student, the manner and ability of assertion and the amount and quality of work taken on board; also being a more mature student and male, people are more prepared to give the respect due to all. It was and is my experience that students are mainly seen as a valuable resource. Most people, me included, like to pass on what they know. As in all human relations it is individuals who make their position within any small group, and their personalities which dictate their relationship with others. (TK/C.82.S)

The academic training and class factors of other professionals were perceived as factors influencing clinical interaction, as this one student reported:

> The position of the nurse/student nurse in relation to other profes-
> sionals is very difficult. Generally, the training other professionals get is
> much more academically based than nursing, and the people they
> attract are generally well educated and usually middle class. Nursing
> has historically attracted people from the working class, not necessarily
> with an academic background.
>
> On the ward we are expected to liaise with professionals and get
> equal respect. This is very difficult considering our different
> backgrounds (and class culture). (BM/C.82.S)

A small proportion of the students observed that their roles were interpreted as either being highly valued or one of rejection by members of the clinical team. This was reflected upon the type of task they were given to do. Here is one example of such a case:

> In my experience this has varied with placements. Sometimes I have felt
> myself to be a valued member of a team and this has reflected itself in
> raising my confidence at what I'm doing. At other times (more
> common) I've not felt particularly valued and it seems I've often been
> loaded with 'valuable learning opportunities' (read: grotty jobs that no
> one else wants to do).
>
> In this way as student you can sometimes seem to lead a dual role,
> one of responsible practitioner when short staffed and another of
> dogsbody when numbers are better or when established staff are in a
> bad mood or not feeling inclined to do much work. I think few staff at
> whatever level of the NHS are, or feel, valued. Most times students
> seem to come at the bottom. (ZR/C.82.S)

Summary of subcategory 4a

The views expressed by a large proportion of students were that, amongst health-care professionals, student nurses endured a low status, and in some clinical environments the qualified nursing staff were also perceived in such a light, this seeming to reflect on the student nurses. In some clinical situations, their views were not valued, whereas a good proportion stated that the perception of student nurses varied from ward to ward, their contributions being valued accordingly. This same proportion pointed out that they were perceived as threats by qualified staff as their knowledge of clinical situations was up to date.

A great number felt that they were respected and accepted as members of the team within the third year of training. It was being proficient in the basic skills and knowledge that gave students confi-dence and credibility. In some cases, being inadequate in terms of knowledge did not influence the level of respect they received from the clinical staff.

A small proportion pointed out that students could create their own position depending on how they projected themselves in the clinical situation. A minority of students expressed the view that the academic base of other health professionals, their social class and their cultural background were factors influencing clinical interactions. These barriers were difficult to break.

The issues raised were:

1. Mental health nursing is perceived as being of low social and educational status.
2. Will a university status alter the situation?
3. Do we have to recruit from different educational levels of achievement?

It is knowing the basic skills and having up-to-date knowledge about clinical situations that gave the students confidence. Their positions and roles on the ward were defined in terms of skills and knowledge.

Subcategory 4b

The majority comments concerned how students could direct their own study if they did not know what to study. They wanted direction about what was expected of them:

Self-directive learning is too demanding. No guidelines, little support. Feel forgotten. I question is it a cop out for School? (BW/D.82.S)

Yes, self direction is FOFO exercises. You can't self direct if you don't know where you are going. (ED/D.82.S)

Self-direction without any direction from tutors is very demanding and uninformative; however with the right amount of direction it can be a good way to learn. (WW/T.K2.S)

The fact that the course was directed by examinations was seen as an indication that teaching staff should keep a certain amount of responsibility for what was expected. This observation was made by a similar number of students, as in the above comments. They perceived self-direction as being lecturers not having planned the lectures, the way out was to propose self-directed study:

Self-directive learning is an excuse for not planning lectures on behalf of lecturers. It requires the student knowing the syllabus from the beginning and covering ground that is irrelevant to the final exams. If there were no pressure to pass exams then this would not be so bad, but while this remains the training will be geared towards attaining knowledge that does not challenge the existing establishment of nursing. Any student who was fully self-directed in the way that certain lecturers interpret would not pass their final exams or be accepted by the nursing establishment. (GK/N.82.S)

Yes, and I also think that teacher-led study keeps a certain amount of responsibility with the syllabus designers – not a bad thing. (DM/T.K2.S)

A small proportion of students made the remark that they only got back what they were prepared to put in:

It depends on how much you want out of things and how much you're prepared to put in. (BK/N.82.S)

No, students, I feel, do what they want to do. If you are interested in something then you'll do work. If not, then you can shirk through the course quite easily. (NOM 11/T.K2.S)

The report from a majority of students was that, although self-direction was very demanding, they benefited from the process in that they were left to work at their own pace. The point that students should accept more responsibility for their study was strongly expressed:

It can be difficult to get yourself motivated at times, but I feel that you learn more if you have to find it out yourself. (KZ/N.K2.S)

I think, yes, self direction demands that a student be highly motivated and yet he/she is working in clinical areas and attending lectures etc. in School where motivation is sadly lacking. How can a student be motivated to learn when she/he is surrounded by apathy? This must be due to the changes in the health service as we know it: clinical staff and nurse tutors are in the middle of change and they feel vulnerable and threatened, and this has a knock-on effect.

On my final clinical placement though, even though the service is undergoing major changes in this area, the staff have been warm and approachable and have encouraged me to learn new skills. I feel that if my group in School had been closer and more motivated we would have been able to get together and learn more as a group. They don't want to learn or to share experiences; they just want to get through nurse training with little or no effort at all. (BW/N.K2.S)

The observations and comments made by a large proportion of the students were that self-directed study was demanding at an early stage. They wanted a form of direction at that stage before they could progress by themselves, a developmental approach with more responsibility towards the end of training:

Self-direction is very demanding in the early stages of training where the actual scope of theory and directions to follow are very undefined. Lack of acquaintance with the service side and theoretical aspects should be addressed initially with a fairly prescriptive, lecture-style approach. The approach which has been followed in our course seems to throw students into an unknown void which seems alternately empty and overwhelming – overall a recipe for disorientation and disillusionment. Self-direction becomes progressively easier with growing familiarity with service side and theoretical aspects. (WL/D.82.S)

I feel self-directed study should gradually become more dominant as the training progresses. I felt I needed some direction to be given to me at first, and self direction was not so much demanding as unproductive. In the 3rd year, however, I think self-directed study to be productive but not too demanding. Maybe if all tutors had a unified understanding of 'self-direction', demands would be less. (BG/D.82.S)

A majority of the 86 students commented that the approach helped them to develop management skills, time management and a sense of responsibility and control towards their education, at the end of which they felt a sense of self-achievement:

No, it helps develop self/time management skills that are required of a qualified nurse. (DM/N.K2.S)

I find self direction quite demanding but as a tool in education it is very valuable as it teaches us to become a bit more autonomous, and I believe this will be helpful to us when we are registered nurses as we should be able to look out for ourselves better. (THG/D.K2.S)

The students felt that self-directed study would not have been demanding if there had been guidance and the climate for it had been created. One of the issues commented on was the mixed educational ability of the group, which affected self-direction. This was reported by a fair proportion of students:

It's not too demanding if the climate is created for it. A total approach of self personal growth and development are the necessary framework, otherwise it is totally out of context and unworkable. (NOM/D.82.S)
Self-directed learning is a very good system if implemented correctly. Students need a facilitator to ensure that they stay on the right track

and to bring them back if they stray too far from the topic. The facilitator was often missing during the last two years of training. (LK/N.82.S)

The comments made outlined how self-direction was demanding in relation to the students' formal education. It demanded self-discipline on the part of the individual, which low morale in the clinical situation did not enhance, commented this one student:

Self-direction is demanding in respect of being totally alien to the formal school system the majority are used to. It also takes self-control and discipline, which can be hard to maintain in the context of nursing with the low morale in the clinical situation, the poor financial rewards throughout and at the end of the training, the lack of respect shown to the nursing staff by hospital management through keeping people in the dark regarding hospital policies, i.e. closures. If these things were redressed I feel sure students would feel much more motivation and in control of their own destinies and have somewhat more to work for, and self-direction would become more of an achievement rather than a chore. (WR/C.82.S)

One student made it known that, in reality, the employing authority dictated what was required, but the emphasis should be on producing what was needed for the workforce:

I think I would have benefited from a more directed course with more emphasis on practice. The best teachers are those who are 'doing the job' and I don't think there has been enough input from these people. After all, should the emphasis be on self-direction when at the end of the day we all need employment and it is the employers who dictate what is required; and if the content of the course is not producing what they want, where do we go from there? (BM/N.K2.S)

The impression created was that self-direction made an increasing demand on both students and tutors. The fact that knowledge was shared with a degree of openness made it difficult for tutors to hide behind the professional organization, and this was seen as a risk that very few were prepared to take. Openness places both students and tutors at the mercy of each other, which was seen as sharing:

My experience is that self-directed learning is far more demanding than directed education but that the value of the learned material is increased in relation to the increase in demands made on the learner. I feel the increase in the demands made on the tutor are so great that very few dare leave the comfort of the classical education system, where they will not have to be constantly alert to changes in the profession, because the ENB will tell them what they need to know.

Experiential learning places even greater demands on both students and tutors, because they have to learn to trust each other and lives are shared, not just the knowledge accumulated during lives.

Many students never manage to open up within the learner group and it would be against all the principles of humanistic interaction to try and force them. The tutors who are not able to make this investment of themselves often choose to hide behind their professional title than even admit they cannot share. (UG/C.82.S)

At times it was demanding, but I think it was up to myself as to how demanding it was, since it was my decision as to how much learning, research, etc., I wanted to do. Sometimes once you uncover something you want to find out more it's not a task but an enjoyment discovering new scopes.

At other times finding the motivation, as sometimes you can, to head on in and burn out the enthusiasm – it's difficult to muster up the enthusiasm to continue. It came and went in hills. But it helped having someone who was enthusiastic in the search of knowledge himself. It was difficult not to take onboard that aura itself. (WO/C.82.S)

Summary of subcategory 4b

The overall opinion was that self-direction was demanding in relation to the formal approach of education that they were used to. A great number expressed the view that they did not know enough about the course in order to direct their own educational needs. The factors they perceived as influencing their training were examinations and projects, which determined how much they should know. Their views were that lecturers should retain a certain amount of the educational responsibility. To be self-directed, students felt that they should know what was in the syllabus from the very beginning of the course.

The view was that self-direction, albeit demanding, helped them to work at their own pace. A majority commented that, from this approach, they learnt more about time/self-management and developed a sense of responsibility and control.

Self-direction was not perceived as an issue by a fair proportion of students as long as they were given guidance and the proper climate was created. One of the problems they identified was the mix of educational achievements of the individuals within the group. An approach to personal growth and self-development was put forward as a framework for training by some of the students.

It was pointed out that the health authority dictated what type of qualified staff they wanted at the end of the day. According to them, the implication was that educational planning should reflect service manager need.

A minority perceived that self-direction made demands on both students and lecturers. What they appreciated in the approach was that lecturers had to take on an open or self-exposed attitude to education: as knowledge was shared, teaching staff could not hide behind their professional cloak. The same proportion commented on the fact that they only got back from the educational system what they were prepared to contribute to the course.

The issues raised were:

1. There was a need for direction from tutors before self-direction could take place.
2. Self-direction should take a developmental approach, with increasing demand on the student towards the end of training.
3. The process involved openness between students and tutors. This was seen as a demanding task for both parties.
4. The process of self-direction needed the proper climate, environment and support.
5. Mixed ability could be seen as an issue in relation to self-directed learning.
6. Self-direction demanded direction, preparation and skill. It was expressed as a form of personal development and self-growth, with responsibility.

Subcategory 4c

Some students pointed out problems of available placements. Their choice was limited because of the shortage of suitable clinical placements that had resulted from health centre closures. This view was shared by a small group of students, as expressed through these two examples:

> Allocation was adequate but at times there was little chance for choice due to shortages of suitable wards. (OH/N.82.S)
>
> Allocation department looms as a nightmarish bureaucracy in my mind, concerned by numbers and fitting people into tight spaces. The element of negotiating with allocations was initially discouraged and then vaguely encouraged by School, although I don't think allocations has come to terms with this. (AC/N.82.S)

The uniform approach of 3 months for every placement across the board was detrimental as it was believed that the length of placement should be left to the skills available in that area. Constant change created stress for students and did not help them to develop nursing skills. Three months, never mind 4 weeks, was too short when it came to developing skills. This was the observation of a large majority of views and one shared by these students:

> I feel that some non-institutional placements are not of benefit to training; otherwise all institutional placements have been of great benefit and very important in preparing you for qualification. I feel sometimes placements are too short in duration. Also perhaps in CFP it should relate more to the qualification (RMN) that you are going for. (CM/N.K2.S)
>
> It is always a problem when getting involved in counselling situations to remember that the longest time a student is allocated to a ward is twelve weeks. In counselling terms this is a short period of time; in psychotherapy terms this can be an instant.
>
> I have discovered the only way to deal with this situation is to 'make this' limitation clear from the outset and make sure the client knows when I will be leaving so work can be done on ending the relationship in time for the end of the allocation. (UG/C.82.S)
>
> It feels that 3 months has been too short for most allocations. It takes a long time to settle into wards and by the time I feel able to perform effectively it is time to move on. Constant change is hard to cope with and very stressful. Most importantly I feel the lack of continuity in the training detrimental to self development.
>
> Three months seems to have been allocated across the board, hardly necessary for high dependency dementia wards or constant observation on CPN allocation; nowhere near long enough for acute ward or elective placement. As for continuity, to have had experience of only one acute ward at beginning of training, followed by general, followed by rehabilitation placement – how can the student possibly develop and follow through any skills? There seems to have been no planning taking into account students' needs; instead allocations seem to fit round the bureaucracy. Also I feel 3 months is not fair on the patient – students pass through and practise on clients, building up relationships that have to be severed when the student leaves.
>
> For staff I feel the length of allocations relates to the above needs of the student. On more intensive wards with more learning opportunities, supervisor and student need time to build up a relationship which they can use to mutually enhance teaching and learning skills. On the more low-key wards a shorter time may be equally as beneficial. Both

...ke patients, must feel uneasy with a quick turnover of students, ...ugh I see students on wards as beneficial for the ward staff, ...allenging and questioning to prevent stagnation and overriding any disturbance in ward routines. (WL/D.82.S)

It was felt that the time spent on each placement should be flexible, being negotiated between the students, the clinical staff and the client. These three students supported a similar approach to the above comments but also requested, for clients' involvement, the service users' rights:

Length of placement, generally allocated 12 weeks. Sometimes too long, mostly too short. Student and client needs not taken into consideration. Should be able to negotiate length of placement with ward team and client. (BO/D.82.S)

Placements have been very valuable experiences but not enough of them have. Some have been a total waste of time and when this occurs the student should be able to change the placement rather than wasting time. (MD/N.K2.S)

The students commented on the fact that they should be informed about the services that existed as training areas. Having a knowledge of what clinical opportunities were available in the placement would be an advantage. This was the comment of a small proportion of students, as expressed by these two respondents:

If by this you mean the involvement of students in working out allocations then it has worked better since I have gained knowledge of what opportunities exist. (MS/N.82.S)

Relationships with allocations have been utilized to give the student as wide a knowledge of the diversity of mental health nursing, to give the student some insight into the differing jobs and roles that they are expected to have. (MC/T.K2.S)

A fair proportion of students pointed out that the time spent in each allocation met their clinical needs:

I have enjoyed most allocations to some degree. Have felt more competent as I have progressed throughout the course and professional relationships have been more effective. (LM/N.K2.S)

In general I have found that a three month placement is about right. A good placement is too short and a poor one too long. It is a fairly reasonable compromise. (NOM./D.82.S)

This one student reported that the value of the placement depended on the clinician and the student, in terms of how they accepted each other:

> Again it depends on who is dealing with the students' knowledge. Some people are willing to accept that student nurses have some knowledge and experiences but others tend to view students as stereotypical 'idiots' who don't have any valuable thoughts and feelings. (G.C./C.82.S)

Summary of subcategory 4c

This subcategory had a poor response in that only 42 students commented, and with limited information, less than for other questions. This might be due to the fact that they might have commented about allocation in other categories.

A small group made the point that there were not enough suitable clinical placements and that they felt as if the allocation services were placing students in tight areas in order to meet training needs.

The feeling that the allocation to each clinical placement was too short for them to feel competent and to build up their confidence was expressed by a large majority.

A sizeable proportion held that there should be flexibility in the type of placement and the time to be spent in each clinical area. These students felt that they should be able to negotiate their placements with clinical staff and clients.

A small group believed that having a knowledge of the clinical facilities that were in existence would help, one student making the point that the value of any clinical placement depended on how its clinical staff perceived the students.

Many saw the placement as being long enough as it taught them how to manage their time in an allocated space.

The issues raised were:

1. Should there be flexibility in the length of placement, depending on the skills available?
2. Should allocation take into account individual students', clinicians' and clients' needs in determining the time on each placement?

How do students perceive their relationship with others in clinical settings?

The object of this category was to explore the interaction between members of different disciplines and student nurses. The subcategories were:

- subgrouping at clinical level;
- the importance of the student nurse support group;
- responsibility as a student;
- the relationship between student nurse and m~~

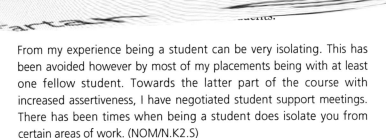

> From my experience being a student can be very isolating. This has been avoided however by most of my placements being with at least one fellow student. Towards the latter part of the course with increased assertiveness, I have negotiated student support meetings. There has been times when being a student does isolate you from certain areas of work. (NOM/N.K2.S)
>
> Does occur, more so when you are an inferior subordinate student nurse. Less so when you reach your third year. People tend to involve third year students more in groupings based at clinical level. It is however a point of demarcation in terms of responsibility and professional definition. (BSC/D.82.S)

A great number of students let it be known that there seemed to be two groups that emerged, students having a tendency to find themselves in one or other of these. A distinction was made between qualified and unqualified staff. This division had an effect as gaining clinical experience depended on which group the students found themselves in:

> The main subgrouping I have found at clinical level is more of a social subgrouping. This tends to have two 'figure heads' and more often than not you are placed into one of these groups by the rest of the staff. This can lead to it being difficult to gain certain experiences depending on which group predominates.
>
> Also, there can be subgrouping between qualified and unqualified staff but this appears to be accepted and even encouraged, especially by the unqualified staff. Also subgrouping between different wards exists; most people think their ward is better than every other one. (GK/C.82.S)

Where subgrouping is seen among the ward staff there appears to be two distinct types. There are certainly groups where the ward staff wish to make a statement about themselves as to how much they want students to get involved.

On other wards there seems to be subgrouping on the grounds that within the ward team it is easier for ward staff to open up in the support group knowing the staff in the group. (UG/C.82.S)

A high proportion of the 86 students were of the opinion that the ward staff often seemed to show dissatisfaction with each other. This resulted in staff being critical, back-biting and being bitchy towards each other. The reasons for the behaviour were not confronted, and this resulted in an unsatisfactory climate for the students in obtaining the required support. Although the nursing staff carried most of the day-to-day responsibility, the medical staff dominated the situation. From their observations, there was no cohesion between the different multi-disciplinary team members. Four students shared this observation:

One of the hardest things I've found to come to terms with in the job. I'm sure it happens in all jobs but it seems more pronounced in nursing than in any of the other places I've worked at. The most important task on starting in placement is to suss out who likes who, and who dislikes who, so you don't step on anyone's toes. I've often looked at the off duty to see which members of staff I will be working with the next day which leads to me developing a cold or not. To sum up, the backbiting and bitching in this job is incredible and it really hacks me off. (ED/C.82.S)

When I arrived on a ward I always found that the staff were in groups of some kind; sometimes the groups were very critical of each other. As a student on placement for 12 weeks I quite often found people were willing to confide in you and sometimes gossip about other groups. I did not really find this a problem because I was able to remain uncommitted to all the groups, since I was there only 12 weeks, but still remain a member of the ward team. (BW/C.82.S)

I have experienced sub-grouping at the clinical level, although this has either been medical staff being distanced mainly by their short time/contact with the ward or student nurses, perhaps in their first or second year actually supporting each other in times of difficulty, such as time for formal support from permanent staff being unattainable due to workload or negatively, I feel as a way of avoiding a simple confrontation of existing practice by moaning to each other about their problems. (JX/C.82.S)

The roles of various subgroups on the ward is, I feel, ill defined. This could be seen positively as the multidisciplinary, flattened hierarchy at work but often it is used as a vehicle for shifting responsibility onto others. Nurses seem to form the predominant sub-group in terms of numbers and often feel themselves to have the most at stake in ward policy. The dominance of doctors, particularly consultants, in individual care decisions, is often resented by nursing staff, who may feel that their direct contact with patients gives them a better perspective from which to make decisions. In my experience, however, doctors are very rarely challenged – partly it seems due to the 'personality' factor. Occupational therapists are generally seen by nurses as more peripheral members of the ward team and are occasionally resented for their greater control over their time and the clients with whom they involve themselves. Nurses see themselves as having to take what comes and deal with the fallout of poor decision making. (ML/D.82.S)

The subgrouping could make them feel an outsider. As these students commented, they were made to feel as interlopers and not given the chance to demonstrate their abilities or talents:

Sometimes the student may be made to feel an outsider or an inter-loper with the permanent staff members who have often formed their own subgroups of either qualified or non-qualified, senior ward staff or staff nurse; they may all go out socially and not include the student in activities, thus not giving the student a chance to demonstrate their abilities and talents. (NL/C.82.S)

The placements were too short to allow the student to be one of the group. The unqualified carers (nursing assistants) saw students as threats to their position. This was seen as an inevitable situation, commented these three students. The feeling shared was that they were also drawn into longstanding disputes:

Subgrouping also occasionally occurs at clinical level due mainly to the fact, I believe, students are only on the ward a short time: other members of staff have a longer time to get to know each other and accept each other's ideas without particularly feeling so threatened. NAs who have been on a ward for quite a while, I have found, are apt to feel their position threatened and their status insecure. (WC/C.82.S)

Do you mean the forming of 'cliques'? In my experience this is an inevitable consequence of working on any ward; probably happens in many other professions too, human nature. Seems to be more preva-lent on long-stay/elderly wards. Can make integration of new staff members difficult. Students can often encounter resentment and hostility from members of staff (particularly nursing assistants) who have been there a long time, especially if the students are very ideal-istic/work-shy/full of new ideas, etc. Easy to be drawn into long-standing disputes when going on a ward as a student; better to keep out of it. Try not to take sides. (BM/C.82.S)

An observation of a great number of students was that the lack of communication between different professionals was reflected in a low level confidence and trust between staff. This led to a hierarchical system as a form of protection and led to a reluctance to join other professional groups. According to these students, this factor affected the training of students and the functioning of the multidisciplinary care team:

I think there is an awful amount of snobbery between disciplines, preventing staff from working together. An element of fear may be responsible but I don't see the rationale behind this. I find this one of the most infuriating aspects of the job and fail to see why it is not tackled by managers responsible. Are people really so unsure of their own value and contribution that they have to resort to this behaviour, and if so why? Having said all this I have seen examples of great co-operation and multidisciplinary work and have also seen the benefits this can bring. (BK/D.82.S)

Having worked on the same ward with fellow students and then alone, I have realized the importance of support from fellow students.

A natural subgrouping occurs on wards and the student finds himself in the middle of what are sometimes raging battles. One of the most difficult scenarios to work under is that where the staff are preoc-cupied with their own particular struggles.

In the MDT, subgrouping occurs in order that each discipline can maintain its powerbase. Token concessions are sometimes made but I have yet to see nurses be given or earn equal status. If nurses are at the bottom of the pecking order, then student nurses are on some plane below that!

After three years there is one group of people who stand out as a group on their own. Of course there are many exceptions and yet the number of angry, bitter and resentful SENs I have worked with is suffi-cient to be able to make generalized comments, in my opinion. Perhaps students pose a particular threat because they are a transient and 'upwardly mobile' group of people, but certainly 'something must be done' about the apparent feelings of bitterness in SENs – more oppor-tunities perhaps? (BG/C.82.S)

They had a need to get involved, commented two students. The support they received came mostly from newly qualified staff, with whom they shared a certain identity. The subgrouping affected the level of students' supervision, and in some cases there was a complete lack of concern towards a certain group of students:

> Subgrouping did occur often on placements; however I felt the need to get involved in both unqualified and qualified groups. (LO/T.K2.S)
>
> There seems to be a correlation between the amount of newly or recently qualified staff on a ward and the degree of acceptance shown towards student nurses. For example, on the ward which I am working at the moment there are two newly qualified staff nurses who have been offering a great deal of support and supervision, which seems to reflect an understanding of the need for supervision as a student learner. However in other areas I have experienced an attitude towards P2000 students which reflects a complete lack of concern for the need for supervision. It would appear that P2000 is perceived as a threat in some areas and in other areas embraced as a progression. (MD/N.K2.S)

A minority of the students experienced clinical situations in which a team approach was in operation:

> Staff mix well; most doctors, OTs, physios, NAs and staff nurses work well together and are part of a multi-disciplinary team. (MN/N.82.S)
>
> Are you referring to students and qualified? If so then the majority of qualified try to involve students as part of the clinical team as they themselves have been students at one time. (NON/T.K2.S)

Summary of subcategory 5a

The feelings expressed by the students were very mixed. A great number made the point that the tension between the different professionals involved in care had influenced their training in that it limited the clinical opportunities they could be exposed to. They saw a large number of the staff at clinical level as being involved in their own power struggle, back-biting, bitching and moaning rather than confronting the issues. They observed a low level of confidence amongst the members of the ward team because of a lack of communication between members of the different professions. The team tended to be controlled by the decision of the medical staff.

The subgrouping created a feeling of isolation and of being inferior, which lasted during the first year of training. The impression students got was that some of the permanent staff felt threatened by them. They were assisted in the clinical setting by newly qualified staff, their main threat coming from nursing assistants.

A small group felt that they were involved at the multidisciplinary team level in the clinical situations.

The main issue relevant to student needs was:

1. What impact did the subgrouping in the team have on the students' training and supervision?

Subcategory 5b

Two students found the group a waste of time as the students did not know how to use a support group. The group was not facilitated, so it tended to be unproductive and negative. It could be useful when students identified a reason for holding the group:

> A group for 'group's sake' is a waste of time. Often in the past groups have been merely negative griping sessions, which only increase depression. However on the last placement we used a group to pass on knowledge and experience as well as for mutual support, and the climate was a lot more creative as well as providing useful support. (NOMI/D.82.S)
>
> I've found that most student nurses don't really know how to use a support group and most student nurse support groups are not facilitated, so I've tended to find that student nurse support groups are usually unproductive and negative. I've found informal support rewarding and productive. (BK/C.82.S)

This one student felt that the group was not supportive as the members were too competitive and thus did not feel comfortable to talk about weakness. This unsupportive environment did not provide the security for sharing experiences:

> My ideas have changed on this as I've progressed through the course. Probably for the first year or so it seemed like a good idea in theory (although I can't say that I found one so in practice). The common bond of being student nurses in a group is not enough security for me to expose my 'weaknesses' by sharing problems with other students. I believe there is a competitiveness between student nurses as there is between other students and I don't wish to give ground to fellow students. (ED/C.82.S)

A support group was not essential, students preferring to discuss issues with their supervisors, commented a small group:

> Student nurse support groups have been helpful but not essential to allow me to ventilate my feelings. Where they have not officially existed I have used more informal lines of peer support or used a supervisor as a sounding board to voice my fears, anger etc. (BG/N.82.S)

Informal support was seen as being most useful as students considered that the formal support group failed to accommodate change. This observation was shared by a minority of the group, as the comments from three of the students show:

> I have not found formal support groups useful; they often degenerate into subgroupings and fail to accommodate change. I much prefer the informal arrangement of going for a pint and a good moan or to take the mickey! (UM/N.82.S)
> Not had an official support group as such, but the general informal support from other students has been the singular most important aspect of completing this course. (AD/N.K2.S)
> I have never felt a need to be part of a student nurse support group. When I have needed support, I have always found colleagues I have selected to be very helpful and much prefer this informal support. From my experience those who seek help from a formal group tend to demand attention and sympathy from all and cannot cope with constructive criticism, and this results in much bad feeling and no support. (BG/D.82.S)

This one student stated that proper support amongst students would decrease the level of sickness and increase the level of motivation:

> It would be beneficial to all concerned with the training as sickness levels may drop, motivation may rise and the level of nurses trained may increase/lower the drop out rate. (ML/N.K2.S)

The importance of student support groups depended on the clinical situation. In some cases, they could be indispensable as a place to discuss things which could not be discussed with qualified staff, who were responsible for writing students' ward reports and level of practical achievements. These three students who shared the above views also stated that the group could be useful for discussing experiences:

I have not actually worked on a ward when student nurse support groups have been operating on a regular basis. I have, however, seen situations where the student group has not been supportive of individual students in ward situations as well as those when the support has been good. (UG/C.82.S)

A student nurse support group can be invaluable, especially if either one or more students is going through something they feel unable to discuss with qualified staff. I often feel it much easier to 'unload' things onto other students as they are my professional 'equals' and they're not writing my report at the end of the allocation. Sometimes the 'them and us' barrier between qualified staff and students can be too big to cross because as you are there for assessment, so you may feel you are being assessed on any negative opinions or problems you may have. (BD/C.82.S)

While on the wards it is easy to feel alone and vulnerable for a short time; supervision is very important but it is not always possible to speak to your supervisor about problems that may occur. Other students may be experiencing the same problems which if shared could be eased, or you may have something to offer a junior student who may feel that a fellow student is more understanding and accessible to them. (PW/N.82.S)

There was a need for support group. For the group to be effective, it was believed that it should be properly facilitated. Students saw the group as providing a platform for a discussion about clinical situations and staff attitudes. They saw the role of facilitating this group as an extended role of the tutors. This observation was made by a large number of students, who also commented that formal support could help in making future groups more cohesive:

Good idea, if they are used properly. Have found that they are attended infrequently and inconsistently. Perhaps would benefit from having proper facilitator. In practice, support seems to take place informally and in small sub-groups, i.e. between students who are working together on the same ward. Think we all need support at some times more than others. Depends on how cohesive group is. Perhaps formal support groups should be initiated and organized from early on in training; get into the habit early on. Good experience on which to base future 'staff support' groups after qualifying. Have found throughout my training that each of us has needed support at one time or another – but perhaps there has not been the facility to give this support effectively at the time; issues have not tended to be dealt with within the group. (BM/C.82.S)

I have experienced various attempts at forming student support groups in clinical situations throughout training. Personally I feel that nurse tutors should be obliged to demonstrate their clinical skills, e.g. group work by facilitating student support groups in clinical areas. In my experience student support groups that are student led tend to be unstructured, non-directive and more akin to a social gathering than a constructive attempt at resolving students' concerns.

The role of the tutor as opposed to a member of the ward staff has advantages. Firstly, much of the criticism and many of the concerns that students encounter on the ward are centred around attitudes of the staff and concern about standards of patient care. The nurse tutor is a neutral participant in the support group process as they have no relationship with either the patient or the nursing team. Therefore any advice would be objective and students would be allowed more openness and freedom of expression.

Secondly, the question of theory and practice could be better addressed when students are debating real situations and events on the ward with the tutor present. Most clinical settings do not object to student support groups, but because of the problems I have expressed, they tend to be formed with enthusiasm at first but very quickly deteriorate because of lack of direction and support. (MD/N.K2.S)

Students found the group to be very supportive, a place where they could share their feelings and offload their emotion, without threat or intimidation. This opinion was shared by a large number of students:

Student nurse support groups I have attended have been run basically in two different ways.

One ward I was allocated to allowed a student meeting to take place once a week but wanted minutes kept of the meeting and these to be available to all members of staff to read. This at first appeared to be slightly intimidating. What was the point of having a meeting specially for students if permanent staff members were looking or appearing to look over our shoulders? The minutes taken of the meetings were a compromise on this ward as it had first been suggested that a permanent member of staff sat in on the meetings, which all the students on that ward at that time promptly vetoed. It was seen that, on the positive side, the minutes communicated the feelings of the students as a group to the permanent staff without one individual having to stand along bartering the group's grievances.

The second student support meeting I attended was a free-for-all, with anything relating to the ward being discussed and a damn good opportunity to get things off one's chest, especially by having a go privately about the ward and its staff members. Not in a vindictive, bitchy way but in a more frivolous, light-hearted banter that eased the stress of a particularly stressful shift or allocation. (PW/C.82.S)

The amount of staff support has varied throughout my placements. However it is my opinion that if the student group have sufficiently 'gelled', then there has always been the opportunity to arrange some time for the running of our own support group, and this has been the best forum for discussing and solving any problems. It always carries more weight if there is a need for change and the whole group is involved, rather than just one individual. (NOM/N.K2.S)

The group was seen as good for sharing clinical experiences and for learning from different sets how they experienced their training. It helped them in confronting ward issues without threat from qualified staff:

A few of the wards put an allotted time aside weekly for student support, run by students on the ward. Its effectiveness is debatable, how effective the time was used; it was impossible for all the students to attend. It is important that such groups exist, if only to ventilate fears, worries, anger, anxieties, to be able to talk them through, and discuss how others handle certain situations; often there are students from different stages of training, along with general students, BA, conversion, etc. and this can be used as a valuable learning situation. (PJ/C.82.S)

I think each ward should have a student support group. On my first placement in the branch programme I had to go on my own to a ward where there had just been a suicide and the staff morale was really low. The atmosphere on the ward was awful; the student who should have gone on that placement with me had chosen not to so I was completely alone with no peer support. I felt really isolated and unsupported.

After a couple of weeks I asked my mentor if I could initiate a student support group and he said yes, and so I did. The rest of the students hated this placement; they had been told they could not have any visits during the allocation, so we used the student support group to change all that and eventually the ward manager agreed to the visits. At the end of my placement I didn't want to leave. I had enjoyed it so much and I'm sure it was because, through the students support group, we had got so much changed. (WD/N.K2.S)

There is a definite need for a support group: this is where the course fell down. I feel that many students need someone to talk to about their anxieties and some way of relieving their stress. I think there should be groups set up for students going through the same things to be able to support one another, instead of trying to get on on their own. (NOM/N.K2.S)

Summary of subcategory 5b

The great majority perceived the need for a student support group during clinical placements. The feeling of being stressed when left in a vulnerable situation was vividly described. Some students expressed the view that they were supported by their clinical supervisor and that the clinicians saw this role of support as being theirs rather than the teaching staff's, a view not shared by other students. There was a hint of lack of trust between the students and the qualified staff.

A large number of students saw the group as a learning situation. They described it as a place in which they could share experiences with others from different groups and years of training, thus learning how to cope with clinical situations. The call that the group should be properly facilitated was made by a fair number of students as they felt that learning how to facilitate the group would make the experience in the support group more valuable for future students.

The issues raised were:

1. Are we missing the chance for community-style learning in mental health nursing?
2. Is the student support group the place for real-life teaching for the nursing lecturer?

Subcategory 5c

A number of students reported feeling that they had very little responsibility. To them, their responsibilities rested with their supervisors or the School of Nursing. Some felt that they had a sense of responsibility towards the clients. They made the point that they were accountable to the mentor, the School or the manager. These two comments reflected a good proportion of student opinion:

> Very little responsibility as a student as they have restricted autonomy, managed accountability under supervision of mentor, supervisors and School of Nursing. (MC/T.K2.S)
>
> I don't think we have to be very accountable to School, ward managers, etc. for our actions. The role of the student is structured in relation to the needs of the ward staff, and tutors take the responsibility for our actions on a formal basis. Personally however I do feel I have much responsibility to the clients I see, and feel I have a lot of power that has to be handled carefully. This can bring about uncomfortable situations for myself, not to mention the client.

> I do feel some accountability toward my employer but don't feel they make many demands. BBK/D.82.S

In some cases, respondents were not sure of their responsibility as a student: it was not clearly expressed; they felt more like a pair of hands. This observation was made by a small proportion of students:

> Responsibility as a student has been unclear at times. Too much I feel has been given to me at times. On the whole, however, I have in certain cases asked for greater responsibility, and I have been given it. I often felt confused as to what roles and responsibilities have been expected of me as a student on the wards. I have often felt like 'cheap labour' rather than an adult learning a profession. But at other times on certain wards I have been able to feel a valuable and productive member of the nursing team. (FM/C.82.S)

A fair proportion of students felt dissatisfied with their training. They felt that students had to take responsibility because tutors could not be bothered to do so, expressing the view that they had to fulfil their training requirements by themselves with no guidance or support. They thought that the level of responsibility allowed depended on how secure qualified staff felt with respect to students. Students felt that the mental health team was just carrying out a patched-up job on the majority of mental health clients:

> Responsibility on the ward/community tends, in my experience, to be something that is 'given' rather than something you can claim for yourself.
> I feel there is a bit of haziness surrounding the legal requirement that you are supervised as a student together with the issue of personal responsibility/liability. It seems to depend on the sense of security amongst qualified staff as to whether they allow you to operate independently under your own responsibility or not. The issue of supernumerary status comes into this as well; frequently where wards are understaffed I have undertaken activities where the issue of my own personal responsibility is unclear. (KL/D.82.S)
> In some ways I didn't feel any more responsible as a third year student than as a first. I certainly didn't feel a great weight in my third year that I was nearing staff nurse. In some ways I feel less responsible. I'm not trying as hard to get things right; a sort of cynicism has stepped in. What are we really doing for anybody anyway? Do people want or are they able to see life differently or more positively? Are we just a patch-up job for the majority of our clients; do they expect too much or do we expect too much of ourselves as nurse therapists?

During my first year I felt an eagerness and responsibility that culminated in feelings of stress and desire to change the world that
sometimes has no basis in reality. (P.W./C.82.S)

Despite the above comments, a proportion of respondents saw their
own status as students as a way out of being responsible for their
actions. They pointed out that their level of responsibility developed
during training. The student banner could be used to avoid any
confrontation:

Easy to abdicate responsibilities as a student using the get out 'I'm only
a student/learner'. In later stages of training, responsibilities placed on
students depend on ward allocated to: some very little. Ultimately the
responsibility for learning and developing is with the learners
themselves. (DL/N.82.S)

Until the community placement it seemed easy not to take any
responsibility, to pass problems to others, but from this time the course
has meant accepting more responsibility. I find it difficult where the
responsibility involves disagreeing with others of greater experience or
higher grade, perhaps acting as patients' advocate – it is easy to hide
under the 'only a student' banner to avoid confrontation. I think you
take on as much responsibility as you want in this later stage of
training; staff are willing to encourage this. (BM/C.82.S)

Students experienced a greater sense of responsibility towards the
end of their training, the second and third years of training being when
they were expected to be assertive in clinical settings. These four
quotes could be taken as reflecting the views of a great number of the
students:

Varying degrees of responsibility, most responsibility when rostered,
during first two years not much at all. Not expected to do much.
(LW/N.K2.S)

It is often said that students have a great deal of power as regards
changing/modifying bad practice in clinical areas. But how many of us
are assertive enough to do this? It is very easy as a student coming onto
a ward for the first time to criticize and find fault with everything. Have
to be very tactful – get the balance right! Ward staff should not be too
defensive and entrenched in old ideas, should make good use of new
ideas, share experiences, be open and receptive.

Placement which I have found most valuable was one in which
I had most responsibility – community. Given my own caseload:
invaluable learning experience. Placements which I have found *most*

demoralizing and unstimulating are those in which I have had least personal responsibility. (BM/C.82.S)

Responsibility is that which students experience as a consequence of accepting autonomy. The ability to take responsibility for one's actions and to be held accountable is one that develops towards the end of one's training and is dependent on the level of knowledge attained by an individual student throughout the training. It is the knowledge of the practitioner that allows the nurse to accept responsibility. (MD/N.K2.S0

Nearer the end of the course we have greater responsibility as we gain more accountability for our actions. (WS/N.K2.S)

The students pointed out that the level of responsibility given depended on their past experience of mental health nursing. They found out that the increased level of responsibility and support motivated them, and this helped to develop their confidence. This view was shared by a large group of students:

Due to the length of the placements in the Common Foundation Programme we were never given any responsibility really, although having said that, on my mental health placements I was given quite a lot, but I think this was due to the fact that I had already worked with two of the staff nurses before when I was a nursing assistant. In fact one of the mental health branch students complained that I was getting more responsibility than she was getting as a branch student. During the branch programme I feel that I have had all the responsibility that I have wanted, and I have taken on more as my confidence has grown. At the moment I have taken on the responsibility of putting together a health promotion/education package with the help of a staff nurse. This is proving to be an excellent learning opportunity for me as I felt let down by the health promotion tutors' input into our group. (BW/N.K2.S)

The responsibility we have had has been different, depending on what ward I've been on and what staff were working. Generally I have enjoyed it more when I have had responsibility so long as I have had good support. (BM/C.82.S)

The ENB make it clear that the student nurses' responsibility is to show they can follow the professional code of conduct. While the student nurses do this their supervisors remain accountable for the students' actions. This had led to a situation where some senior nurses seem to want to prevent student nurses taking any responsibility for patient care even in a supervised role.

This I find unfortunate because, reflecting on my training, I am aware that I have developed more as a nurse in the situations where my supervisors have allowed me to take more responsibility for the therapy, be they directly supervising the session or supervising me following an individual session between the patient and myself.

As for student responsibility towards the learner group, how this is taken seems to me to vary greatly between students. The majority of students seem to me to be far more responsible in their dealings with patients than they do in their dealings with fellow nurses.

One area where students and qualified nurses alike appear less responsible than I believe they ought is that of confidentiality. It seems an acceptable practice to discuss patients on social occasions in a way which I feel breaches confidentiality in many cases. Perhaps this is a result of nurses not having the facilities to support each other in a more appropriate manner. (UG/C.82.S)

A small number expressed the opinion that their responsibilities consisted of being motivated, keen, ready to learn and to confront. The 3 years should, according to one of them, be viewed as a privilege, and responsibility should be earned rather than given:

I feel my responsibility as a student is to challenge, confront and question. This is only just becoming easier for me as only now am I beginning to feel competent to do so. I still tend to keep my thoughts to myself. I hope I can improve on this. I also feel it is a student's responsibility to be well motivated, keen and ready to learn; I feel we should feel privileged to have 3 years' training when we have little ward responsibility and should not abuse our own self responsibility as students. I am also aware of our responsibility towards clients, both in helping and supporting them, in being respectful and tolerant. (WC/D.82.S)

Throughout my training I have felt responsible for my actions, but I feel that others need me to have experience, e.g. become a third year student nurse, before I am trusted. I've found that if I've earned the respect of senior nursing staff then I am allowed to take more responsibility; when I haven't earned respect then I've been not allowed to take responsibility, which seems fair enough. (BG/C.82.S)

These two students' comments were that responsibility rested with the care team and the supervisors:

In the clinical area it is negotiable as to how much responsibility one feels happy with, i.e. key-worker or co-key-worker with client, with the nursing team. It is a personal choice with a student as to how much one wants to accept. I have never really thought about my responsibility as a student; I have always been involved in team nursing and jointly responsible with other team members to plan and implement all aspects of care, team meetings/ward rounds with the MDT. It has always been a team effort. (EK/C.82.S)

Yes any client requires the best we can offer and that I feel is my responsibility as a student. If we don't do this we might not be irresponsible but we aren't working to the highest standard we can. I also feel a responsibility towards my supervisor for his/her accountability for my actions. (NOM/D.82.S)

The students' sense of responsibility related to themselves, to how they wanted to develop as individuals. Their commitment and responsibility was seen as parts of their own personal development. These four examples expressed the view of a majority of students:

Does the UKCC professional code of conduct cover students?

It was my responsibility to gain/develop as much as possible and it was my responsibility to behave in a way that promoted well-being.

As to being responsible for others' safety and care this was primarily in the role of observer and passing on information to qualified staff as well as maintaining a safe environment. (JX/C.82.S)

In what I see as a maturing process, I have learnt that I am not as responsible for clients as I originally supposed. Self-defence plays a role. The gusto with which I first embarked on therapy was unsustainable and also unrealistic. I was taking on responsibility for clients, not realizing how harmful this can be.

Personal responsibilities have greatly increased: more children, greater commitment to 'non-work' activities, have caused me to question the level of commitment that I can offer to clients. I will now set limits and be brave enough to implement them. I will not be afraid to say 'no' as I see this as therapeutic in itself. (KP/C.82.S)

I have always been given responsibility while on placements, sometimes much more than usual. Other facets of responsibility are related to the course, management of your own study time, etc. (CM/N.K2.S)

You are responsible for your own learning, i.e. seeing the opportunities and taking them. And also responsible for your own conduct. You have to be responsible enough not to accept too much responsibility. (BAC.KA.LO./C.82.S)

Summary of subcategory 5c

A great number of students pointed out that the level of responsibility increased with their stage of training, a greater sense of responsibility being enjoyed in the third year. The level of responsibility allowed depended on the placement and how confident the clinical staff felt about the student.

A good proportion of students, albeit accepting their level of responsibility toward clients, pointed out that the ultimate responsibility rested with the School of Nursing and their clinical supervisors. A minority used their student status as a camouflage and as a reason for not confronting clinical issues. A small number of students made the point that they were being used as a pair of hands, whereas others perceived it as a privilege to be in a learning situation and felt that this should not be abused; to them responsibility was to be earned.

A large number saw themselves as being more responsible to their clinical supervisors or the clinical situation in which they were involved than they were towards their fellow nurses. A sizeable proportion of students expressed their dissatisfaction with their training and viewed students' responsibility as an opt-out for teaching staff in meeting the needs of training.

A large group pointed out that their level of motivation and confidence increased with the level of responsibility given and the level of responsibility they were prepared to take. Responsibility and commitment were perceived as elements of personal development by a majority of the students.

The issues raised were:

1. Were students responsible for doing or for knowing?
2. Do students gain confidence and motivation from doing rather than knowing?
3. Are teaching staff responsible for their knowing and clinicians for their doing? If so, what is the role of the students; do they have shifting responsibilities as a result of their student status?

Subcategory 5d

Three-quarters of the research groups expressed the view that hospital managers were unclear about the students' role, the relationship between manager and student being close to being non-existent. This could put the students in a powerful position as they felt the School to be answerable for their actions:

Student nurses seem to have an ambiguous role. They are occasionally supernumerary, occasionally expected to make up the numbers with the responsibilities entailed. I feel it important that our role is made clear. Management, in my experience, has had little control over me as I have always felt autonomous and self directing, accountable more to the School of Nursing rather than ward management. This puts students in a privileged position which they can abuse. I have made positive use of the freedom this has given me, though it can at times be limiting as to what you can or cannot do as a student. (WL/D.82.S)

I feel that the relationship between students and management is an area that could be greatly improved. I think that management sit in their ivory towers and don't know or understand the needs of a student nurse. They don't understand the needs of a patient so what chance has the student got? (BW/N.K2.S)

Students' only contact with management was to make complaints and to take part in the evaluation of the clinical placement. These two views reflected a large number of such comments:

Do not feel, for myself, that there is much contact between students and management. Do not feel that I am known to management as an individual. Managers meet students for an evaluation at the end of each module, but this tends to be very superficial. Not sure whether our needs as students are really heard and respected by management. Do they act upon what we say? They should do because students can give valuable feedback about each clinical area. (BM/C.82.S)

Relationships between myself and management distant. Only contact is when complaints made. Very little exchange of information. (BG/N.82.S)

Students made a distinction between different levels and types of management, seeing both good and bad models. The overall impression was, however, one of distance and indifference to student needs. They stated that managers were working in isolation from the clinical areas and had little respect for or knowledge of the clinical situation:

My experience of the management of the School of Nursing is that it is as poor as the management of the mental illness service as a whole. Both sets of managers appear to me to be power hungry and officious, yet they try to hide this behind a facade of egalitarianism and concern for the people they manage. This is shown no more clearly than the way they seem to move staff around without at any time consulting individuals of their wishes and in total disregard of individuals' skills.

This contrasts sharply with the effectiveness with which some ward managers I have come across motivate their ward staff into providing the best care in often difficult situations just by showing genuine concern and respect for the individual nurses.

I challenge any claims that this is not possible with hospital management because of the size of the venture to look to industry where a number of very large companies vastly improve their industrial relations by having a more integrated relationship between managers and shop floor workers (the Nissan factory at Sunderland, Co-operatives, information from TV documentaries, I cannot remember which ones). (UG/C.82.S)

Contact with management has been minimal over the years. If ever I have met a manager I have never felt they are particularly interested in me as a student, sometimes to the point where you are not even acknowledged. At times I have found I have little respect for those I have met, as they just seem quite isolated from the ward and its problems. Just to clarify, with management I am talking about senior nurse upwards. However, no manager I have ever met has stuck in my mind as being exceptionally good or not so good. This I put down to the lack of contact. As a student I have never felt considered in any managerial decision for a ward, this being exacerbated by permanent staff on the ward who seem to think you don't need to know and you don't have an opinion on the subject. Even if you say otherwise. (BG/C.82.S)

This was very poor in CFP, feelings of insignificance. Only in the last placement have I felt that my opinion has been taken into consideration and not felt self conscious. (NOM/N.K2.S)

Although the relationship between students and managers was poor, the following students felt that a good relationship was essential for change to be implemented. They still believed, however, that managers were detached from clinical areas:

Very poor; we are the last to hear of any changes and often the first recipients of change. A good relationship between students and management is essential if any kind of change is to be implemented against the current mode of non information. (ZL/D.82.S)

As far as I could see there is no relationship between the students and management. The management make unilateral decisions and expect the student nurses to comply with these decisions. (GC/C.82.S)

A large proportion of students pointed out that ward managers and course tutors were the point of contact and that they were supportive.

The respect for ward managers (charge nurses) was expressed by most of these students:

> I don't think there is a relationship beyond ward management and that has been supportive to the learning experience. (BL/C.82.S)
>   Apart from the course tutor, I feel that little or no encouragement was given from the School and management. (BC/C.82.S)

Summary of subcategory 5d

Students perceived managers beyond a certain level as being poor or isolated from their needs. Thus, a greater majority made the point that managers were not aware of the students' role; the only level of manager they acknowledged with respect were tutors and ward managers.

The issues raised were:

1. If that was how managers were perceived by students, did they need to consider their role in training?
2. The comments and expressions used by the students were very strong and supportive with respect to ward managers but very critical towards other levels of management. How could this issue be addressed? Should managers take a more active part in teaching and clinical work?

What effect does training have on the students?

This category explored whether encouraging assertiveness in the classroom influenced the clinical experiences of students. It also explored the effects of training, the rules governing training and finances on the students during the 3 years. The subcategories were as follows:

- self-assertion in the classroom/ward;
- anxiety/fear associated with training;
- finance/social position and reward;
- ground rules and safety during training.

Subcategory 6a

A large proportion of students made the points that self-assertion depended on the personality of the students and that no amount of practice or presentation would help towards its development. It grew with confidence, aided by practice placement and with some form of theory before practice. They also argued that longer placements would help in building their level of confidence:

I find this difficult to comment upon as assertiveness is a topic which seems to have been missed throughout our training. Some sort of theory is needed before practice in the classroom environment. (AL/D.82.S)

I think that this depends mainly on personality and no amount of lessons, practice and presentations will ease or teach this to people who do not have a wish or inclination to be assertive. I think it is wrong to push people unless they've expressed a wish to but it is something that grows with confidence, which would be aided by longer placements. (LW/N.K2.S)

Although assertiveness was considered to be a personal issue, an equal proportion felt that it was easier to toe the line and play the student role on the ward. Moving beyond this attribution could make their situation uncomfortable. It was easier to be assertive in the classroom than in clinical placements; a good ward report was more important than challenging clinical staff:

Self assertion is a very personal thing. Not everybody is naturally assertive. Is being assertive for a naturally reticent person also a role? It depends what role you see yourself in: i.e. staff see you as student and you behave accordingly. Some may feel more assertive in the classroom rather than ward or vice versa. Sometimes assertiveness is not appropriate and this is also dependent on reflecting on past experience. (BAC,KA,LO/C.82.S)

Self-assertion on the wards differed from ward to ward. Staff on some wards appeared threatened by self-assertive students, and staff on other wards welcomed it. Overall, in spite of how liberal staff onwards might be, there was still a tension which I can only guess at being that students should tow the line. But I don't consider this to be totally wrong – there have to be certain limits and rules on every ward for them to function. (KB/C.82.S)

The same proportion of students made a similar point, but they also experienced a degree of discomfort when confronting ward staff. The classroom culture, with peer support, was seen as being supportive and encouraging self-expression, but the situation on the wards was different:

On the ward some staff nurses looked down on students and if they spoke out they were seen as bolshie. We were often not allowed in staff support groups to voice opinions on the ward. Comments such as 'you're only a student' or words to that effect were often said. (LC/N.82.S)

The classroom provides quite a safe environment to assert yourself in, especially if you're not particularly used to doing this. However it took a few months for me to feel comfortable with this. On the ward self assertion is a whole new ball game. Sometimes it is encouraged by staff, which at first can be quite disarming. Some staff reinforce your subservient student role, a role at first I was more than happy with due to the lack of responsibility. However after working on a ward in the 2nd year, which very much encouraged assertion, I found it very frustrating on subsequent wards where they still expected you to behave like 'a student'.

I found it very hard to respect these people, who I felt were holding me back more for their reasons than my own, that they felt quite comfortable in the 'power' of being a staff nurse. When challenged about certain issues I found these people invariably 'backed down' about how they viewed my role but then they made comments about 'my attitude' behind my back. Luckily, these occasions have been rare but it can still be hard work, if not to get people to listen to your viewpoint, to take that viewpoint into account when making decisions concerning you. (BG/C.82.S)

In my view the concept of self esteem (as I understand it) is a predominant feature of psychiatric nursing in general and the training process. This stems from the interactional nature of the job, a constant dynamic between self and others, a low incidence of orientation to task. This arises both in School and on the ward but there is some variance in my experience of self assertion in the different areas.

The atmosphere for assertive behaviour can feel 'safer' in the School context in that views may be supported by a number of peers. On the ward, however, disagreement and complaints may bring one into conflict with an entire ward culture, leaving one to be ostracized by most staff members. Perhaps this is more of a fear than an actuality. The classroom is clearly an area where one can learn to put one's views across without fear of recrimination, whereas on the ward I feel a more delicate course has to be steered when putting forward views, steering around different conceptions of mental illness attitudes to patients and characters.

I don't feel that the experience of assertiveness in School particularly helps one to be assertive on the ward, and the two environments are fairly divorced from one another. (GD/D.82.S)

These two students believed that peer pressure played a part in developing assertion, this meaning in some cases who shouted the loudest. They felt that respect from others helped to develop their skills. To them, assertiveness implied power, self-directedness and trust:

This is a very personal area as all people assert themselves in different ways and to various degrees. The factor of peer pressure in the classroom has a major effect on self assertion as some are always able to dominate and put their view loudly. It is up to individuals to make their own path if they choose. After all, to be able to function well on a ward you must be prepared to assert your view but with respect for others. (BG/C.82.S)

How the student perceives those around them plays the biggest part in how assertive they choose to be. My experience within the classroom is that of being able to trust those with me to accept me as myself – all my classroom experiences have taught me our class is a relatively safe place. The times when the class has not been safe tend to be related to either trusting visitors more than they warranted or when group members made mistakes of which they were truly sorry.

Ward situations are different. I have perceived that the staff on some wards are so set in their ways that I would feel uncomfortable in challenging them beyond a certain point. My experience on one ward was that voicing 'officially' what everyone had complained of when we discussed the matter got me labelled a troublemaker and that this attitude made me worry about how therapeutic the ward could be with staff of that type.

On other wards my critical input has been sought, as the staff were aware that 'new eyes' can often see how to improve a poor situation that the ward staff did not realize existed. (UG/C.82.S)

Two students said that self-assertiveness skills could be transferred from the classroom to the clinical situation. Their views were shared by a small number of others:

Self-assertion learnt in the classroom is useful on the ward but I still find manipulation is more effective. (LT/N.82.S)

Generally, mentors and ward staff are receptive to assertive, enthusiastic students because it implies a certain degree of willingness to learn. Assertiveness is important in self-directed learning as it is often expected that students will direct their own learning needs by request. In P2000 training in particular I have found that the extent to which students are assertive directly determines the structure and quality of the learning experience. The implication of this is that the non-assertive, passive learner may not gain the maximum involvement and participation in a ward or negotiated learning environment.

Self-assertion in the classroom tends to be directed around debate and discussion of issues, theories or in role play. This environment can be a place where the student can develop his/her assertiveness skills, although the goal is often to put over a point of view rather than negotiate for individual learning objectives as one would on the ward. (MD/N.82.S)

Two students presented opposing views. The first felt threatened in classroom situations, whereas the second one related the relevance of the classroom to practical situations. The knowledge skills and confidence built during project presentations were seen as being transferable to the ward:

For me the classroom is an unsafe environment. I think that the group has never worked together or shared as I thought we might have at first. I have always felt insecure and vulnerable in the classroom, which is a shame because if it had been a good group we could have all shared our experiences and we would have grown together. On my clinical placement, where they take a group approach to care, I am at the moment in a psychotherapy group. This is proving to be very painful for me and it would have been beneficial to bring this to share with the group in School had they been the supportive type. (WD/N.K2.S)

To be assertive in the classroom and on the ward has to be a goal of any training. How it was achieved for me is a result of a combination of things; to begin with I had my previous knowledge and confidence, which was developed through a process of or similar to graded exposure.

The value of project presentation in developing self assertion cannot be underestimated. Being able to present verbally one's work and beliefs to the group, being relatively safe and on the whole receiving positive feedback, enhanced each individual's confidence. This confidence in oneself permeates throughout the rest of our lives, for example, ward rounds, case conferences, etc., where the passing on or discussion of information requires confidence and composure, attributes which can only be achieved by hard work in collecting and analysing information using relevant theories and belief in one's own capabilities, a respect for others and a conscious use of self or own feelings and experiences being valued. (JX/C.82.S)

The views expressed by the following four students differed from those above in that they felt that a broader-based knowledge and wanting to listen could build their confidence and made them feel comfortable. These views were shared by a majority of the group:

Self assertion both in the classroom and on the ward comes with a broader based knowledge of both theory and practice and the confidence to express these under the scrutiny of other health care professionals. People have differing interests and may feel confident about expressing ideas on one subject but may want to sit and listen to other people's views on other subjects. (PW/C.82.S)

As self-assertion has developed for me on the wards, so has self-assertion in the classroom. The two seem to go hand in hand. I find assertion difficult and I think we need assertiveness training workshops at the beginning of training. (WB/D.82.S)

Obviously some people are more assertive than others, but I have found that being assertive stems from the fact that the individual is confident, and this confidence is gained through having knowledge in what you are doing and the ability to express yourself. I think the experience of classroom seminars has proved useful in boosting an individual's confidence, particularly if the group in which these discussions/seminars have taken place have been comfortable and non-threatening. They can also be a source of motivation.

Assertion on the ward is more difficult, even if you have the knowledge at your fingertips; it is hard for your views to be accepted, particularly on short placements. The longer the placement the easier this is but again lack of experience and student status do not help individuals who are trying to be assertive: no matter how much theory you know your lack of experience is obvious. (BW/N.K2.S)

Summary of subcategory 6a

A great majority believed that assertiveness consisted of both knowledge and practice. Developing oneself in the classroom through discussions, seminars and project presentations assisted in being assertive on the wards, but some students said that their assertiveness skills came from practice rather than theory.

One of the issues pointed out was that not all clinical staff are comfortable with assertive students. Being assertive placed the student in a difficult role; they felt that it would be better to play the required role according to their role attribution on the ward. A good ward report and achieving the required practice level of clinical practice on a placement was seen as more important than being assertive on the ward.

A small group made the point that assertiveness meant respect for others and being confident in oneself. Some others perceived manipulation to be as effective a style of communication.

The issues raised were:

1. How could the ward and School situations be brought closer to minimize the level of discomfort in both students and clinicians?

2. Would presentation of seminars and case study discussions at clinical level by students, lecturers and clinicians help this issue?

Subcategory 6b

The greatest level of anxiety was caused by having to face the unknown, becoming a staff nurse and gaining employment. The feeling of a leap into the unknown was expressed by a large number of students and well summarized by these three:

> Training is very anxiety provoking especially in the latter months. There are no provisions given to deal with any anxiety and stress; therefore I feel that 'burnout' is increased by this. (CW/N.K2.S)
> Anxiety and fear related more to being qualified, leap into the unknown, etc. (WW/T.K2.S)
> Anxiety – fear associated with training. With the new P2000, anxiety and fear re training and future employment have increased dramatically, along with frustration – low morale and general bewilderment. Fear of unknown throughout training. What next? Being unprepared for new wards and constant upheaval of tutors caused anxiety – not feeling of any value within School of Nursing. (BB/D.82.S)

Moving from place to place needed adjustment. The theory–practice gap was felt to be an open issue. These issues, together with the unknown element of the clinical situation, affected a majority of students, poor communication between staff increasing the tension. These clinical situations, tied up with course requirements, for example exams, could make the situation unbearable:

> I feel the last three years have been very anxiety provoking, initially fear of not knowing what was to happen throughout the course, then jumping from ward to ward constantly meeting new people in new surroundings and never really settling in anywhere. Now anxieties about exam results and job prospects – very worrying!! (LT/N.82.S)
> There is a certain amount of anxiety provoked purely by the unknown element of new situations. Also an anxious client can provoke anxieties in professionals working with them. Everyone starts to run around in a flap and nothing is achieved. I think in that sort of situation you need to develop a clear sense of your own personal boundaries and role so that you don't get sucked in. Going back to the unknown element – due to poor communication or misinformation, a lot of things are 'unknown' to the student needlessly. (NOM/D.82.S)

Don't fear training – I do fear qualifying. Anxiety at times is unbearable because of bad time management of the course; you can have assignments, exam and placement all at once and at other times nothing. (CL/N.K2.S)

A large proportion of the 86 students commented that mental health nursing was a reflection of their own life experience. Having to face some of the issues in others that they did not want to face in themselves created the most anxiety, but at the same time having to deal with these issues in others helped them to become a more able person. Here is one example:

I have found that throughout my training I have encountered very anxiety provoking situations but have faced (most) of them and come through them OK and learnt quite a lot from the experience. I think this reflects real-life where we all have to face situations which we don't like but as a result of coming through them have more experiences and more towards becoming a more able person. (WD/C.82.S)

These students stated how the feeling of fear experienced at ward level could be uncomfortable but at the same time challenging. These four examples show the diversity of this experience:

I had many fears and anxieties whilst doing my training and before I did it. I had left a safe job and took a reduced salary, so I had fears in case I could not manage financially. The person who interviewed me knew me from the wards and said that he didn't think I was academically good enough to complete the course, so this was another worry. I am a very shy person and it takes a long time for me to settle in a place, so I had many fears about the endless 4 week placements where you just get to know people and then you had to leave. I hated having to be observed doing a task and I found that tasks I had been doing for years on my own I now couldn't do without making a mess of them. I hated speaking in a group, and each resolution week in the Common Foundation Programme caused anxiety provoking situations for me; I was always glad when I had done my presentation, one because it was over and done with and I could relax and enjoy the other students' work, and two, because it would have been so easy not to come to School and miss the week like so many of our group chose to do, and I didn't. (DW/N.K2.S)

Objectively, I feel that my confidence has increased during my training. I feel that group experiences in School, by providing the continuity of a group in which I could feel increasingly more comfortable to discuss issues, has been a contributory factor. Presenting projects and conveying information to the group has changed from an extremely anxiety provoking experience to a slightly uncomfortable but quite challenging one. This has allowed me to feel more confident when addressing groups in multi-disciplinary meetings, handovers and so on. (SW/D.82.S)

I have encountered a great deal of anxiety during my training – mainly through lack of confidence and relevant experience. I have often felt completely lost and overwhelmed by so much going on and so much to learn. I have also felt very self-conscious on wards, especially when observed by supervisors. My fear has been expressed through anxiety. I have never felt fear at, for example, threatening behaviour, violence, etc. (WL/D.82.S)

I do feel that a fundamental anxiety I have had about my training is my difficulty empathizing with the apparent need for so called objectivity in both my clinical practice and assessment, as well as an ideal for nursing. I disagree and feel awareness of self (one's own beliefs/attitudes and how they affect one's responses) and respect, understanding, and rational discussion and an open mindedness are of greater value than the detachment and pseudo professionalism that objectivity has displayed throughout my experience. (JX/C.82.S)

On a new clinical placement, students could feel apprehensive at first but also supported by their supervisors. This factor helped to improve the situation. This point was made by 10 of the students, of which the following quotations are two examples:

There is apprehension on commencing a new ward. If there is real fear then either there is no adequate supervision or the person needs to evaluate personally why fear should exist. (IK/C.82.S)

Always fears about the unknown but when I have been bothered about something and admitted it, support has been there from mentors or other staff members. (CL/N.K2.S)

A large number of the students pointed out that the level of anxiety decreased with time and with group support, although clinical contact could still be perceived as threatening. Acute care placements were seen as the main source of tension and anxiety:

Each ward (or the prospect thereof) brings anxiety of a greater or lesser degree. Just the constant change every 3 months is upsetting to one's routine. Perhaps you have established a certain role in a place only to have to start again. One ward may treat a 3rd year with respect and as a person, then you are catapulted into an environment where your opinion is irrelevant and you are seen to be incompetent.

Initial anxiety was high since I had not had any contact with 'mental illness' in the clinical setting. First clinical contact (KLB) was of the high point re: stress levels. I threw myself in and was burnt out after 5 or 6 weeks. I was given responsibilities beyond my coping abilities but with hindsight prefer this way of learning: 'in at the deep end'. I made several howling errors in terms of people's sensitivity and pain – true I have learnt from this but was it too painful to the person on the receiving end?

Only now do I realize the anxiety that I, as a student, posed to qualified staff. Present styles of teaching encourage a close group – three people from such a close group going into your working environment must be a considerable threat.

Was I prepared enough for each allocation or the initial experience? Well – this is difficult to assess. I see myself as having been very immature in the way I work about things, as much as more mature – doubtless in 2 years' time I will see my present stance as rather foolish or immature. It might be foolish to look back and say this could have been different or that. I was different so what I find appropriate now I probably would not have done then. I must say I feel that I should have been brought down to earth rather than lifted to heady idealistic heights. This might have led me to be more gentle and sensitive in my approach. (KR/C.82.S)

Anxieties include – fear of violence before first acute allocation, a fear perpetrated by introductory block tutors. Fear over examinations, which I think is natural and to some extent important. My particular anxieties in my training occurred most markedly in terms of the tremendous stress during my speciality placement on an acute ward. Stress for student nurses, particularly in acute areas, is simply not properly identified as an issue. (BG/D.82.S)

Summary of subcategory 6b

Students believed that their training was stressful. As one student put it, they were involved with real-life situations and with having to face through others what they evaded in their own lived experience. The most stressful factors were course work, examinations, having to change clinical placements at short intervals, fear about their ability to perform adequately following qualification, fear of employment at the end of the course, and in some cases fear of clinical situations (e.g. violence). Acute care placements were seen as the most demanding clinical experience.

A large group stated that their level of confidence increased during the course, but the fear of examinations, assignments and changes of placement regularly reared its ugly head. A small group felt that they were supported by their supervisors.

The issues raised were:

1. There is a need for support during clinical placements.
2. Clearer directions are needed to limit distortion in communication.
3. There seems to be a call for student support groups, or a kind of support, because of the demand made on students.

Subcategory 6c

To this one student, his financial situation was disastrous and he was being kept by his partner:

> Financially disastrous – I would not have done the training if I had not been kept by my partner throughout the training. Working on a ward has given me a social standing because even as a student you are treated like a 'professional'. Amongst friends there is a mixed feeling from one of adoration to dismay at what I am doing. I decided that after 15 years in a job I did not like I would do something that I wanted to do, so this has to be a gain, but whether I should be discriminated against financially because of this is another matter. (KV/N.82.S)

A majority of those who took part pointed out that pay was bad during training and low after qualification. They felt as if they were being used as cheap labour and were uncertain about getting a job:

> Money is very poor at first and not that good in the end! I'm not aware of any difference in my social position apart from losing dole status! It feels good when people ask what I do though, and the rewards are really to do with what personal satisfactions you get out of the job and also the increase in confidence that it has given me. (BE/C.82.S)
>
> I came into the nursing profession primarily for personal satisfaction, although the financial rewards were also a consideration. However, being a mature student I had the experience of working in other areas and as a result have been able to make comparisons. I have worked for the Post Office, the Health Service, in a clerical role and have been a shop assistant, and I can honestly say that I have never felt so undervalued. The 'dedication' of nurses has been abused for too long. In no other profession would you be expected to work later than your set hours and not receive either recognition or payment for it.

With the closure of many NHS hospitals and setting up of Trusts, many of the old contracts have finished, which has seen the requirement of more flexibility of nurses to do nights and unsocial hours. There is also the threat that they will lose their power of negotiation over pay, so that not only will they be dictated to about the hours they work but also the pay they receive. The scales are being tipped even further when considering the new skill mix, i.e. few qualified staff with more responsibility and great accountability but with no extra money, support or recognition for it. I feel the status of the qualified nurse is being gradually eroded.

The final 'nail in the coffin' so to speak has been the fact that, after completing 3 years' training, there are no jobs available with only a guarantee of a 3 month contract of 16 and a half hours per week. There have even been doubts about the ability of Project 2000 nurses to do the job!

Another reason I was attracted to the job was that I envied the opportunities which nurses had to learn. Obviously it is an essential part of their job to continually update their knowledge, but with the continual cost-cutting in the Service, access to courses is difficult and funding has become another burden for the conscientious nurse. MD/N.K2.S

Social position could be seen as a good reward, even though the job was not financially rewarding:

I think I'm biased because I have 3 young children so it seems to me that for a single person the social position and rewards are pretty good. However due to social security ratings we are at present in a poverty trap; e.g. the 3rd year pay rise made me £10 a week worse off! This led to having to work a couple of evenings in a bar, decreasing time available to study or spend time with my family and causing tiredness, etc. (NOM./D.82.S)

I have struggled with finances whilst on the course and I have found the travelling expensive. However, I do think that it has been worth it. (LE/C.K2.S)

Because I have never had a well paid job I have found the wages in nursing present no problem to me. They are adequate for my lifestyle. In society most people regard nurses with warmth and admiration, and I have found that when I have met people and told them I am a nurse their reaction has been different. I'm not sure how I feel about this. I know I like to work hard and like to be thought of as working hard but I don't like the 'angels' image and it has nothing in common with me. (BW/C.82.S)

The following three students did not perceive the financial aspect as a problem. They felt that helping someone and being acknowledged for doing so was very rewarding. They also felt the training gave a realistic expectation of life:

> I do not feel my salary to be that low; yes, in comparison to a postgraduate salary, but in comparison with jobs I have held before and similar jobs I could get elsewhere, my wage especially now as a 3rd year I don't think is too bad. I have to be very careful with money but I don't consider that to be such a hardship at this time of my life. Perhaps if I was older with more responsibilities I would think otherwise.
>
> Social position I consider to be quite low, partly due to some negative attitudes of the public towards psychiatry, partly due to being a 'male nurse', which is still a shock for some, and partly due to being a 'student nurse', who by many seem to be considered irresponsible 'youngsters'.
>
> I feel the rewards can be quite high in spite of the bad days when you do feel dreadful, but the reward is from actually feeling you have done something positive for somebody else with positive feedback from both staff and clients. One of the main rewards I have got from doing my RMN has been getting to know myself and gaining a much more realistic outlook on life. (BG/C.82.S)
>
> I have found no difficulties with financial situation – probably because I have no ties or responsibilities. I have managed to pay for several courses in my own time. (WC/D.82.S)
>
> Not a major consideration really. Personally I have found a student nurse's pay sufficient given that quite generous benefits are available. At a time of writing this I have a net wage of just short of £10,000 p.a. when benefits and poll tax rebate are taken into account, and this does not include unsocial hours. Social standing for nurses is high. Banks and other finance industries look favourably on such guaranteed professions (or so I am told!!). Not really a problem here. (RK/C.82.S)

Summary of subcategory 6c

A good proportion perceived the financial reward as being adequate, although the great majority said that they did not feel rewarded for what they did and the responsibility that they undertook. The perception of the status of nurses in the public gaze was mixed, with judgements of both low status and good status.

Subcategory 6d

The students felt safe amongst their peers but exposed at the ward level. The major concerns for most of them were safety at the clinical level, issues surrounding the communication between staff, and the staffing level. The same proportion felt that the College treated them as children:

> I feel within the student group there is no sense of vulnerability, but perhaps we have just reached an optimum level of disclosure and don't venture beyond it. Concerning safety on the ward, I feel staffing levels and poor communication often undermine a sense of being safe, and one can feel exposed and without adequate fall-back, particularly for example in speciality situations. (CL/D.82.S)
>
> I have always felt safe on wards and College, and ground rules are relevant, however I feel that College can be too dictatorial and treat students like children sometimes. (LW/N.K2.S)

The views expressed were that certain students abused the situation and got away with doing nothing. These views were shared by 20 of the students:

> Ground rules have been blatantly abused by certain students, and as the group has not been very close knit, people get away with doing their own thing. On the whole general safety is kept to a high standard. (DT/N.K2.S)

This one student said she did not feel safe, but nobody wanted to rock the boat:

> Very good idea but don't always work. Safety in nursing doesn't exist because if the boat is rocked nobody wants to know, never mind support you; e.g. sexual harassment is rife, abuse of patients, complaints about the course, e.g. *Nursing Times* letter. (ED/D.82.S)

The rules provided a safe place within which to explore their feelings, said 12 of the students. Although the ground rules were flaunted on several occasions, the level of honesty kept the group culture alive:

> The ground rules established by M87 gave me, once they had been proven, a safe place to explore ideas; although they were often flaunted and eventually smashed, they paved an opening for me and to a degree, formalized in a positive manner our work. The illusion of safety was comforting and needed by me. With M87 I discovered something new. Three safe people whom I could totally trust; this more than anything else gave me freedom to grow. (GS/C.82.S)

I personally felt glad about ground rules being set in the group. I'm sure this had some bearing on the conduct of the group even though they were broken on numerous occasions. I feel sure that when the rules were broken seriously the people concerned reflected on the consequences of their doing so and it had an effect on their conduct for the rest of the period of training.

Although some members tried to take over the group I'm sure this was seen for what it was, an attempt to boost a fragile ego or some members being naturally open and more willing to discuss their ideas and possibly more confident in front of an audience.

Ground rules will always be broken but there must always be an open and honest facility to discuss the repercussions and feelings this might evoke. (PW/C.82.S)

Summary of subcategory 6d

A great majority felt that the ground rules provided a certain level of safety for exploring their own feelings. There was a certain feeling of lack of trust toward the School and the clinical situations being expressed. A large number of students expressed the view that some of their peers abused the situations in order to get away from doing any work.

One student expressed the feeling of being abused. The support obtained in that situation was considered by the student as being limited.

One issue raised:

1. Should there be a learning contract between students themselves and a contract between students and lecturers.

Chapter 8

Group discussions and student reflections

The data from the individual accounts, outlined in the previous chapter, have been detailed and have provided a vivid view of the lived experience of training. In this chapter, commentaries on the audio-recorded discussions will be presented. I have decided upon this format of presentation in order to prevent a repetition of what has been presented in Chapter 7. This discussion largely confirms what has already been stated so is a kind of triangulation on the individual accounts presented. It has added advantage in that it gives an indication of how the students related or did not relate theory to practical situations, and it gave in some cases a taste of how the students experienced practical situations. This relationship to practice, and the manner of experiencing practice in supervised situations, has been vividly described by one of the students, CC/5.82.S, the account giving a very clear and well-written description of the experience of training (see Ramsamy 1998).

The presentation of the commentaries, on discussions and reflections, will take the following form:

1. May 87: group discussion and reflections – 12 students;
2. May 88: group discussion and reflections – 12 students;
3. October 88: group discussion and reflections – 16 students;

During the commentaries, I will be relating to the appropriate group and making references to specific students in the group using the same system described in Chapter 7. Each group commentary will use only the initial of the student's pseudonym as the groups are identified, those who took part following the 82 syllabus. A selected account of the discussion of each of these groups can be found in the appendices in Ramsamy 1998, and these are used to support the commentaries. The appendices are arranged in the original thesis as follows:

- May 87: Appendix 1
- May 88: Appendix 2
- October 88: Appendix 3
- Drop-in centre: Appendix 3A
- Acute care: Appendix 3B

May 87 group discussion and student reflections

This section comprises:
- the group approach to teaching;
- the effect of training on self and others;
- how relevant the experiential approach to training is;
- group feelings.

Group approach to teaching

The group was made aware at the very beginning of the course that the course would abide by the ENB training regulations. Being a professional course, it was also subject to the professional Code of Conduct set by the UKCC, and being employed by the health authority, it had a contractual responsibility to the employer. To these were added the ground rules for the group. These were: respect for self and others; giving each other time and space; not being judgemental about what others expressed; speaking for oneself from the perspectives of one's own experiences; not making generalized comments; giving feedback to each other; commitment and responsibility in one's actions; and providing confidentiality to create trust.

This style of work gave a structure that facilitated the students to become aware of their feelings and 'their ego defence mechanism' (ZX and XY). It provided them with a good foundation in how to deal with situations in the clinical setting and made them aware of their counselling skills (ZX and XY). The discussion gave them an awareness of a group approach to therapy in the clinical setting. During the discussions, the environment facilitated self-confrontation and the clarification of what was happening and made the students aware of the damage that group members could do to each other.

XH expressed his dissatisfaction about the way in which the group rules came into being. The ground rules encouraged complete freedom of expression, but freedom with responsibility. According to JX, there was no negotiation regarding the ground rules; the students felt that these rules were not theirs, although they used them and the rules served their purposes in that 'what the ground rules serve were a sense of belonging' (JX). At this point, XY took the opportunity to say, 'I remember one incident from you sitting in that chair over there looking, and the ground rules, you actually said that these, the ground rules, are not just words which made me feel being confronted.'

HT felt that the group was 'quite firmly structured', although the two initial facilitators of the group were different in their approach. The students felt surprised at the rate at which the group activities moved, and they 'still feel a lot of positive things in it'. In the process of linking what took place in the classroom to the ward situation, RK commented that the group 'experiences take me away from the group to ward situations'. This view was shared by CC, who stated that the group helped 'to control your fear and anxiety and helps you recognize that'. CC 'felt annihilated' and it 'throws me back' as the group developed; 'It was like forming a relationship with patients. In that way it has helped me in ward situations.'

According to VI, who came from a small village, the approach helped towards personal development and 'working in the group ... was utilized on the ward'. These views were supported by BG and HT, who made the point that the group approach stopped them patronizing others. It stopped their judgemental approach, and they gained from this. According to HT, 'it was sit and talk and listen. Examine my own views with a supportive environment and people I really trust which is something of a novelty to me.'

VI expressed a feeling of intimidation at the barriers that had to be overcome within himself. A feeling of openness was created by trust, which broke through the barriers, but 'there was no feeling of therapy and being told how to deal with it'. VI wanted direction but felt that words were just being bandied about, 'words like empathy, trust and confidentiality'. The fact that only some of the students lived together in nurses' residence exacerbated the situation in that the group discussion carried on after classroom activities for these students. Now the feeling was that there had been no trust at all, 'there was no true confidentiality'. VI felt that the group moved too fast.

JX agreed that 'we destroyed the facility we created or that you created'. XH made the point that it was a learning situation, that there were many positive aspects arising from the group and that a lot had been gained at a personal level. BG stated that 'I came here and accepted responsibility' but felt compelled to take part through group pressure. JX shared the same view as BG but made the point that no direct pressure had been exerted. PW joined in and tried to clarify the issue by stating that there was a feeling that not being part of the culture 'was in some way less than enlightened, some way inferior', but agreed that 'looking back that was my responsibility', to take part.

From the above discussion there is evidence that:

- the group was aware of group dynamics and of the level of deception that could take place in a group;
- the relationship to practical situations was made from the classroom to the ward situation;
- the individual gained from this approach in terms of personal development and interactive skills;
- although the ground rules were questioned, they benefited from the safety and trust or mistrust created.

Effect of training on self and others

This issue has been touched on in relation to group teaching. In dealing with the above issue, there was a general feeling of anger in the group as they felt that, as far as getting a job was concerned, it was 'on a road to nowhere' (JX). Although the students felt good about their training and that it 'has been exceptional about my personal development', they felt robbed, 'used' and (JX) about being not sure of gaining employment in the area.

CC, who had been a silent passenger through most of the course, made the point that, compared with the general training, this course was different: 'I did not have any confidence when I started and I am talking now.' CC was tired of arguments in the group by then. The utterance from CC silenced the whole group.

At this point, KG accepted that, because of the lack of limits imposed, the students revelled in the situation in which they found themselves; 'it was an environment for which I myself and a lot of people were not equipped'. XY talked about facilitation: 'I pretended and conned people. I pretended I can facilitate that and challenged you.'

HT made the point that the group activity influenced their whole life: 'the past six or seven years were poured out'. JX said that what was experienced was that 'for the first time in education or in work situations, I felt that what I can produce was important but I, as a person, was important'. What was uplifting about the group was that 'we were important people'. The feeling expressed was that the safety in the group was alien to the outside world, 'the harshness of reality'. The students did not consider their faults, and this left them with a false sense of safety.

Here again, the issues of personal development and trust/mistrust are raised. The point made very strongly is that such a group may deceive itself in the false safety of its own environment. These issues are part of the psychodynamics of the group, in which one member may use language to impress others, the motive being conscious or unconscious. What is important was that the pretender gained insight into the causes of his or her behaviour for the journey has to be made.

How relevant the experiential approach is to training

Some students made the point that it was sometimes important to perform in clinical situations without the use of their personal experience, acting like an 'automaton' (JX) or approaching clients using 'humour' and 'superficial chat'. Seeking permission for tasks helped to 'get round the intimidation' of clients; XY saw this as a kind of caring.

XH felt that the first 3 months of the course were a form of caring. This was perceived as a time when the students could realize the importance of their own experiences in creating an awareness of their situation. The discussion was broadly based but related to a topic relevant to their experiences. The presentation of specific topics by the students generated their specific pain. Talking about themselves around a topic 'helps to expose the pain' (JX). To them, these situations acted as both therapy and education.

Working in that style with projects, experiences and presentations produced a knowledge base. This made 'the clinical situation more meaningful' and gave individuals a feeling of importance; in so far as they knew what they were doing, 'the experience' was used 'as a yardstick' (JX). This form of experience with awareness helped to prevent a transference of feeling from themselves to the clients (XH). At this point, XY revealed that it was the 'stigma that I caught up about my past and over-reacted', and the agreement was that experience was seen as useful when used in a positive form.

The discussion then moved back to their anger towards the School and the fact that they were not allowed to organize a trip to Bradford related to a day workshop on transcultural psychiatry. They eventually made the trip under their own steam on their day off.

The point made in relation to an experiential approach was that it was seen as an embodiment of skill, knowledge, interaction, emotion and a form of action. The students believed that personal experience could be confronted through project work and with the style of presentation described above. The experience gained through this style created a kind of self-power – 'your experience is the yardstick' – in interacting with patients; it created awareness. This might help to prevent transference during interaction. Caring as described was not intense therapy the whole time but concerned with the more mundane aspects of life, such as humour.

Group feeling

The experiential approach generated an intensity of feeling, as described above. The point made here was that to be able to use your own power, you have got to know your client: 'do your research about your client, you are respected' (XY). The students pointed out that negotiation could only start from a point of power. The way to become an autonomous person was seen as being directed in what to learn, a chance of getting a job afterwards; these were the factors that encouraged negotiation and the style of facilitation (JX). The knowledge and confidence gained during seminar presentations and this style of work helped in developing an 'ability to confront and assert my views in the open' (JX). To XY, it gave confidence for self-expression in case conferences. These were the steps to self-power.

Respect, courage, safety and knowledge were the aspects that were seen as helping to develop self-confidence and assertiveness. The experiential approach was seen as an embodiment of self, a tool, a 'yardstick', that guided oneself during interaction with others.

May 88 group discussion and student reflections

The topics here were:

- experiencing support from the group;
- the anxiety associated with training;
- the responsibility to self and others.

The group of students wanted a support group to discuss how they were experiencing their training. Their aim was to reflect on how supportive the group had been and how it had developed from the start of their training. From the beginning of the discussion, the tension in the group gave an uncomfortable feeling, with an air of restlessness and agitation. The density of the group environment was such that it could be sliced with a knife. It was as if they had had a discussion between themselves before calling the group. This was when the element of support/non-support was recorded.

Experiencing support from the group

The students wanted support from the others within the group, but it was not forthcoming. Although they were supportive towards each other at the beginning, they seemed to have lost the potential 'to offer it, but for a certain reason we have lost it' (XI). They had stopped talking about their feelings. 'We sat down doing the evaluation', we discussed 'how we feel about supervision and how we feel about being on the ward, were objectives met' (XI), but we 'don't talk about our own feelings' (XI). This observation of needing support was acknowledged by NON, who stated that 'this is certainly the most difficult job I have ever done. You need some support from people who are doing the same thing'. This comment silenced the group for an intense few seconds.

XI then let it be known that they were not the only ones going 'through this thing' and made the point that some were receiving outside support and that they could not transfer the support to the group. MX made the point that support was given by individuals within the group and that it was unrealistic to expect group support whilst on clinical placement. This comment generated a feeling of anger in NON, who initially called the group and commented that the 'group was not that closed anyway', and NONII: '[I] have lost interest in coming to School'. The anger could be seen: 'so just leave it, the whole job is rubbish'.

The group support and the subgroup support developed during the course seemed to have evaporated, with a feeling of lack of trust; as BW pointed out, 'I certainly would not disclose anything any more to the group ... I would choose certain individuals.' The change in the group seemed to make 'you feel like strangers to the other individuals, which I think is quite sad' (BW).

NON re-stated the point that they did need support and that 'you can't get it on the ward ... they are not students', even though they might have gone through it in their time. To NON, 'as long as work goes I think people in this group know me better than anyone, anyone on the ward'. If the group could not give the support, 'we might as well call the whole ...', 'I don't know whether people want it to be anything or not. I am just fed up with it. I don't feel comfortable, the way it is' (NON). The students thought that the introductory block (the beginning of the course) was 'pretty difficult'. The change, which was gradual, had left them 'not feeling happier at all' (NON). At this point, NON felt that the support from the group was not forthcoming and spelt out that 'some people may not be bothered about it, that's why I suggested it. I did not want it to be me having to do all the talking.'

The students pointed out that this was the most difficult job they had ever done and that they needed support from each other in the group. But the support was not forthcoming. This led to a fair amount of anger and pain for NON. They felt that their feelings, and how they felt about their training, did not seem to matter much. The central point of discussion seemed to concern evaluation, when they were questioned about ward objectives, clinical supervision and their feelings of being on the ward. In a sense, the concern was about the mechanics of education.

Anxiety associated with training

The concern expressed was, 'am I doing the right thing or am I doing it wrong?' (BG). They felt that they had never been advised by 'someone on how to do counselling on the Ward. What are the different stages, how to get the counselling "situations" (BG). Learning was derived from the patient and they knew they had been of help when the patient said 'you have been helpful'. They were told to have a care plan without an explanation of what to aim for in delivery of care.

'There must be a structure as to where the patients are being moved when they leave the ward' (BG). At this point, LI spelt out that 'I have not got my point across. I know where everybody goes. I don't know whether I am doing the right thing.' The feeling was that the students did not know whether they were doing the 'right stuff' when they were with the patient for an hour. At this point, LI spelt out that they were not sure 'whether the theory meets up with the practice. Theory–practice not made clear.'

This discussion illuminated the difficulty of linking theory and practice that the group was facing. This difficulty provoked a certain amount of fear over what they were doing whilst caring for patients. They seemed to take their guide for their level of performance from the patient's reaction as they were not sure how to apply the theory, for example of counselling, in a given situation. The instruction relating to the care plan was not clear either: they were told to have a care plan, not knowing what to aim for. This group wanted a clearer direction for the educational input and how to apply theory to practice situations.

Responsibility to self and others

The concern about responsibility was seen as a kind of contradiction in that they were told that, as third-year students, they had control, but now the message seemed to be that 'you have not got responsibility, you are not qualified'; as you are an outsider, 'not the set working on the ward', you cannot be given the responsibility' (MK).

The point made by three students at this stage was that whatever was said by the ward staff did not matter, for 'when you are with a client that's when you are in control; there is nobody actually standing on your shoulder saying you will do this, you will do that'. The patients 'see you as a nurse', 'whether you are trained or not' (SU, LI and BK).

According to SW, the patients saw them as having power as a nurse regardless of 'whether you know what you are doing or not'. EX raised the question of whether this kind of responsibility was 'authority' or confidence, to which MX replied that you just used what you had learnt before and acted according to the situation, accepting responsibility for what you did, although MX was not sure 'whether I would like the responsibility'. NON pointed out that the ward staff had more confidence in 'me than I have got in myself' and that 'I don't mind asking anybody patient or staff what to do.' BK's reply was, 'that's how we learn'. 'Yes with added pressure', answered NON. To be left in charge, not knowing 'what we are doing' (MX) is worse when 'we are third year'. To be told that they have got first-year students on the placement and not knowing what to expect left them feeling that 'I am there but I don't know' (XT). This state of not knowing was also observed in the qualified staff (NON).

The discussion then moved on to the fact that medical staff and the hospital manager had got control over finance and resources (BK). MK made the point that quality of care depended on the attitude of senior nurses, to which MK stated that, when there had been a shortage of staff, 'I tend to be treated more as a qualified nurse' and then 'back down again', which created conflict in oneself.

The students felt that pressure was being exerted on them by their tutors (NON). They pointed out that they were treated as tutors' 'babies' and without the right to select their group tutor (MK). The group stated that they could do with some supervision (EX). BG replied was that they wanted reassurance, along with some direction of what to do and someone confronting them in what they were doing.

The group pointed out the following issues:

- Responsibility was a kind of control that they were given because they were third years and was then taken away because they were not members of the ward staff and not qualified. At one stage, they were seen as able for being third-year students, whereas in the next instant they were relegated to being of low student status. They perceived this action as resulting in conflict in their role.
- The students felt that they had power whilst they were with clients regardless of whether or not they knew what they were doing.
- They pointed out they did not feel confident to be left in charge of a ward.
- The group expressed the view that there was a need for supervision, which should be confrontational to make them reflect on what they were doing.

October 88 group discussion and reflections on supervised practice

This group had taken their state final examinations six months earlier. The six months during which they had been waiting for their registration had been spent as student nurses under supervised practice. Each of these students had a supervisor for the period awaiting their registration.

These accounts will be presented as follows (see the Appendixes in Ramsamy 1998):

- the drop-in centre project
- the acute care placement
- a personal account of supervised practice (CC/D82.S.; see Ramsamy 1998 for this account).

Drop-in centre

This project was for establishing a drop-in centre for psychiatric patients and for any members of the public who wanted some support in their daily life activities. It was undertaken by three students: BG, MX and LU. Their aim was to provide a day facility different from the day psychiatric centre in that anyone could walk in freely and the activities would be whatever they intended them to be. These activities would be organized jointly by the three students and those attending. From their research on qualified staff opinions, they knew that there was no interest in this kind of activity as there was no professional value attached to it: occupational therapists, doctors, social workers, community psychiatric services and art therapists did not see any professional glory in this type of work.

The three students felt that there was a need for anxiety management, group therapy and so on. What was missing was 'actual friendliness'. They set a place where ex-patients or members of the public could have the opportunity to do things that professionals tended to overlook, activities such as music – playing records from which conversations could be initiated. Some of the conversations could be quite intense, for example, talking about medical diagnosis and medications, or they could be as ordinary as talking about dogs and cats. The major problem the students identified was that the patients or ex-patients had problems in finding someone to go out with socially, and taking on this task in such an informal setting demanded responsibility on the part of the individual.

The three students presented a paper to the nurse manager, the project being financed for three staff nurse salaries for a period of one year. Seven years later, the day centre is still serving its purpose, and professionals have started recommending that their clients attend it.

What these three students displayed were:

- the ability to assess the needs of the clients or patients;
- skill in setting up a system to meet those needs;
- the research skills to justify a need for the centre;
- an ability to convince the nursing management of the need for such a service and to get the project financed, displaying an excellent application of knowledge to the practical needs of a community.

Acute care placement

The three students involved in this were BC, GL and ED. They acknowledged their limited knowledge of medications and were prepared to seek help during the six months. Their concerns were the dosage of medications, prescription, the side-effects of drugs, the administration of medications and the sections of the Mental Health Act. They were aware of the integration of drug administration with nursing care and the relevance of knowing about the medication in order to educate the clients.

Care planning

The students were involved in caring for a client who had attempted suicide by trying to hang herself. After the incident, she was taken to an intensive care unit, where she was unconscious for a few days and was given a 25 per cent chance of surviving by the medical staff. Following her recovery, she was transferred to a psychiatric unit with her newborn baby. Whilst in the intensive care unit nearing recovery, her care plan had not involved one-to-one observation. On her transfer to the psychiatric unit, the care plan aimed to prevent self-harm as she had attempted suicide a few times; she was thus placed on a one-to-one observation to prevent her from harming herself and her baby.

The students found the care plan difficult to implement. They only way to deal with the client when she was disturbed was to 'strip every-thing out of the seclusion room and lock her up; that's the only way to deal with it'.

According to the three students, it was very difficult to practise what they had read in books. They had to pick up some skills, then read about such a situation and then get feedback about their action: practice followed by theory and feedback. The way this group learnt was thus to get on with the task, learn whilst on the job and then question their actions in relation to a theoretical perspective, getting feedback from others, including the patients.

A personal account of supervised practice

This account (by CC/D.82.S, Ramsamy 1998) is very descriptive and personal, revealing the inner feelings associated with learning. This student was highly involved in mental health; to her, mental health training was the development of the self, which could be seen in her individual account. This account has been selected for its vividness and fluidity. The emotion generated in it portrayed the crossroads between knowing and doing or not knowing and doing when faced with a particular clinical situation.

Discussion of resarch data

In reviewing the history of madness and of caring for madness, I pointed to the contrast between the 'scientific' approach, which relied upon physical intervention, and the personal developmental approach, in which an emphasis is placed on self-responsibility. In view of this, it must be said at the outset that this contrast was not an issue for these students in training. There is no mention in the research data of any difficulty in how these students cared for their patients as a result of their having to serve two different philosophies.

The problems facing students arose from a number of sources, but the uncertainty in their role did not appear to come about because of a perceived conflict between attending to physical treatment and caring at an interpersonal level. These students accepted that nursing requires an integrative approach and were more concerned about the practicalities facing them in concrete situations than about any philosophical dispute.

This concern might be a later-appearing reflection, but in any case its absence does not imply its insignificance. The possibility remains that it is the absence of an integrated and explicit philosophy of caring for madness, which gives due respect to both the physical/impersonal and the personal, that lies at the root of many tensions in the profession. We will return to this theme in Section III.

The major issue that arises from the research data is perhaps the students' concern for bridging the gap between theory (the knowledge of the academy) and practice (the skills required in clinical situations).

At one stage, the students made the point that, as a nurse, one needs to be thrown in at the deep end in order to learn about how to handle clinical situations. This comment was made repeatedly by a majority of students, who argued that it is only by being confronted with different clinical situations and reflecting upon the experience with the help of a supervisor that learning occurs. Having the support of qualified staff whilst practising was seen as helping to develop a degree of confidence. This supervision and reflection on practice is viewed as the way of bridging the gap between theory and practice.

The clients/patients were seen as being a necessary focus for the transition from theory to practice. Through the process of identifying with clients, the students developed a feeling of concern for them. By sharing and discussing the experience, they gained the respect of clients. As some students put it, when a patient says, 'Thanks very much for the chat yesterday', then you know you have assisted him or her.

Some of the groups were very critical of the teaching staff in the School of Nursing. They were seen often as a hindrance rather than a help. There were, however, a number of cases of students expressing the view that researching and presenting projects in seminar sessions to their individual student group helped to build their confidence and self-respect. Also, during multidisciplinary team meetings, and indeed within clinical situations, they developed the confidence of talking in groups and could relate clinical incidents to projects undertaken. It was felt that, for this skill to develop, an open approach to discussion and feedback should be encouraged.

The other major factor that assisted in bridging the gap was the student support group and informal student groups. Student support groups were highly valued by some, but not all (see Ramsamy 1998), of those who attended them. They expressed the view that, by a full discussion with other students who were at different stages of training, they learned how to handle the clinical situations with which they were dealing. Students expressed fear and mistrust when qualified clinical staff wanted to have the meetings formalized and recorded. A large number of students pointed out that student support groups would benefit from being chaired by teaching staff. They also pointed out that it would be easier to learn by working alongside their personal tutor.

The issue of theory and practice was expressed clearly in the account of the last six months of training from the October 88 group (see above). The account of CC/D.82.S relating to supervised practice gives a vivid account of how one student perceived supervision.

Being supervised whilst practising makes a lot of demands on the students. Reflecting upon that experience was what helped to build confidence and self-power. Self-empowerment of the student was seen as a practical, developmental issue, linking knowledge, ethics, emotion and action in clinical situations. A good example of this is provided by the group who established the day facility. This development clearly needed a great many skills, which these three students displayed. The group of students concerned were qualified when the project was undertaken (as they had taken their final examination six months early) but still under supervision.

Although some students commented that it could be best to hide under the role of 'a student' when faced with a difficult situation, the overriding view was that students need to take responsibility and have the confidence to use their practical, experiential knowledge in clinical situations. The gap between knowing and doing could only be overcome through such an initiative.

The relationship between the student and the supervisor was seen as being critical in helping the student to link academic study and practice. A supervisor was seen as somebody who provided the 'bouncing board', the 'arm-band' and the 'life-line' for practice. The level of confidence and respect between supervisors and students was perceived as being the main ingredient of the stock of their relationship. In this practical world of nursing, the students pointed out that they would prefer to have a say in who their supervisor should be rather than having the selection or matching being carried out by the ward manager. A group of them made the point that they wanted somebody with whom there was mutual trust and respect.

Learning in clinical setting was, as we have seen, influenced by peers, clinical staff and the clients themselves. Some students perceived themselves as being of low status, belonging to a different social class from other members of the multidisciplinary team. They also perceived themselves to be used by permanent staff (ward staff) in situations of tension on the ward. In some cases, members of other disciplines tended to be too guarded about what the students knew. That students could also hide behind their identify and role was expressed by some. Their role as a student nurse also affected their relationships outside training, a small minority stating that they kept their private life separate from their student one.

The anxieties that students experienced related largely to the demands that mental health training made on them. It was described in some cases as going through personal development in the full view of others, and as one of the most difficult jobs that one was expected to do without support. On the whole, the students felt a lack of direction. Having to be self-directed with no guideline on what was expected left the students feeling bewildered. They expressed the need for a structure or framework. Self-direction was perceived by the students as a 'cop out' by some teaching staff. Those in the group who possessed a structure for how to organize their learning, for example BG/D.82.S, L/5.82.S and BG/N.82.S, benefited.

There was also some anxiety relating to finance. There were mixed feelings: although nursing was perceived as being financially unrewarding, it was felt by some that nurses were valued for what they did. The financial aspect was perceived as an individual responsibility in terms of its management. That the formal and structured approach to education that they had experienced influenced their learning style on the course was clear; coming from a teacher-led style of education, most of the students found the transition to less structured forms of learning difficult.

In relation to the major concern of this thesis – the use of experience in practice – the students felt that there was a need for a structure to help them to arrange their practical experience in a way that made it compatible with the plan of training.

Summary

The research data suggest that the task of relating experience to effective practice needs some form of structure. Although students recognized that their learning must inevitably consist of an immersion in the practicalities of clinical situations, with all the attendant uncertainties ('being thrown in the deep end'), there was also much confusion in terms of which direction they were going in. There was support therefore for a structure that could co-ordinate the input of the teaching staff, the student, the clinical setting, which includes the supervisor and client, and the theory.

This mediation between these different facets could be seen as one which could only ultimately be put into place by the students themselves under supervision. This supervision, in turn, required an openness on the part of both student and supervisor as some of the students perceived mental health nursing as their personal development.

In the following section, the issue of how to address the mediation between personal experience and a structured education will be investigated. An account of the relevant research literature in mental health nurse education will be addressed, followed by a raising of the possibility of putting forward a philosophy of care for mental health nursing, with specific concern with the pre-registration course.

Footnote

In this section, the data presented arose from two different syllabuses: the 1982 syllabus and Project 2000. It is not the intention of this research to clarify the difference between the two. Instead, the aim is to look at the use of experience in caring for patients.

There are obviously some differences in that the Project 2000 students commented on their shorter allocation in clinical areas and their perceived lack of skills in dealing with clinical situations. They put this down to the fact that they spent only 18 months in the mental health branch and that, out of this, there were only 1000 hours of compulsory clinical experience. This shortage in the length of place-ment was also commented on by the 1982 syllabus students, although they spent the full three years in mental health. Both groups made use of the same clinical facilities on mental health placements, and their supervisors and lecturers were from similar backgrounds. The textbooks and social context of caring were also similar.

The differences, as already stated, lay in how the syllabus was struc-tured in terms of content presentation and in the form of theoretical assessment and examination. One of the bones of contention between the two groups was that Project 2000 was graded as being higher acade-mically (diploma level), whereas the 1982 syllabus course was credited at 120 points at Level 1 certification. The other concern was that Project 2000 students were not placed in the same clinical areas as the 1982 syllabus students, although the supervisors for Project 2000 were trained under that syllabus.

Section III
Developing a philosophy

'The only reality that exists for an existing
individual is his own ethical reality. What would be
the use of discovering so-called objective truth, of
working through all the systems of philosophy
.... to construct a world in which I do not live
but only hold up the views of others'.

Kierkegaard, S., (1835), Journals

Chapter 9
A philosophy of mental health nursing

A Philosophy

This book, and the thesis on which it is based, has tried to show how the past has influenced the present, in the hope that it can contribute to the future planning of the caring process. On our journey, we have gained an understanding of how different traditions perceived madness and managed their situation in relation to caring and the use of experience. How the different elements or parts of the caring process have been articulated with each other to form the Gestalt of care has not been a smooth and consistent development; instead, we have seen both continuity and contradictions.

The contradictions focus around the issues of control and treatment along the lines of the medical model versus the development of personal autonomy and reflection. This holds true for both carers and cared-for. We are, in a very real sense, confronted with the opposing philosophies of the person, the one empiricist and mechanical, the other stressing personal freedom and autonomy.

The purpose of this third section is to propose a philosophy of caring that can do justice to the experiences of carers and patients and thus serve to ground the practice of psychiatric nurse training. It begins with a further examination of the lived experience of the students in training, relating these to the recent research; this leads onwards to a model for a developmental approach towards reflective practice.

This section will take the following format:

- The critique of caring
- Developing a philosophy for mental health care with a developmental approach towards reflective practice
- The way forward.

The critique of caring

This critique will take into account:

- Nursing and caring – the lived experience of students
- What does recent research tell us about theory and practice?

Nursing and caring – the lived experience of students

Our account has shown that the students' experience of caring in the field, which involved the wards, the community and the classroom, has been one that demanded involvement and commitment on their part. This field, which was made up of the supervisors/mentors, lecturers, patients and different professionals, was where these students developed the skills and knowledge upon which their perceptions of caring and being cared for were formed.

The different regions from which the perceptions of caring were developed each carried their rules and regulations, without which understanding the perceptions of caring would be anything but caring. It is the traditions or sedimented knowledge and the rules that authenticate caring. Within these regions, just as the different professionals were involved in their tasks, so too were the students also involved, and it was their embrace of these traditions that gave them certain attributions and status, thus defining their role.

Roles and attributions will be dealt with later on in this section. What concerns us here is how the tradition of continuity and contradiction, as described earlier, still influenced the students' perceptions. From various comments (see, for example, NON/C.82.S), caring was the most demanding job the students had ever done, and it was described as one in which they needed support from those 'who were involved in the job'. What they wanted was support and reassurance; what was offered to them were questions on whether the educational objectives had been met, whether the clinical supervision had been satisfactory and how they had got on on the clinical placements, all concerned with the mechanical aspects of the course. What these students wanted was support from their group. What we offered them in return was a mechanical feedback process. We are dealing with students with an average age of 30–35 years, the youngest being 18. They were involved in an area in which very few dared to venture, and their needs were met with contradictions. We were so warned by Connelly (1856) and Batty (1758), who were worried about their attendants being used and abused in order to save money. Are we now concerned about our mechanical educational principles in dealing with the mental health nurses whom we care to attend to or educate?

The other aspect of concern was the tensions, conflicts and frictions the students came across during the process of caring. Caring, a demanding task, became a paradox in learning how to care. Students had to be exposed to the conflict between the different regions and the tensions between the different professionals in the caring field. From the data (category 5, subcategory a), we can see that students were involved as go-betweens between the different professionals and permanent staff in cases of conflict, a role that made them feel powerful. In this caring field, where they learnt from the patients and enjoyed their mediating role between the permanent staff, there were feelings of fear and anxiety about caring for patients on acute admission wards. Caring thus involves a fear of the others and mediation in cases of conflict.

The relationship with the mentor/supervisor was not always a clear-cut one in that students felt they could not confront him or her as a good ward report was seen as a better option than confrontations about certain issues. Others felt comfortable with their supervisors (see category 3, subcategories b and c).

The role of these students must be seen in the context of the ward, as the space through which the students 'transported the message', in Goffman's phrase, had a profound effect on the meaning of their social and learning situation. In some cases, these students had specific rules applying to what they were allowed to do. Some felt like pairs of hands (category 3, subcategory c). Others expressed the view that they were given responsibilities or were seen as being responsible when it suited ward staff (category 5, subcategory c). In their learning 'occasions', their time on the placement was limited, with high and low involvement depending on how the ward staff predicted their level of participation.

Goffman argued that every situation or learning opportunity of the student must be viewed against the 'backdrop' as the 'message' does not travel in a vacuum (1953, 134). The social context played a great part, and this depended on the 'participant' status. The level of 'euphoria' or 'dysphoria' would depend on the mode of message that the students carried with them on the ward (Goffman 1953, 240).

The role of the students could also be confused by the students themselves with their own form of self-deception. Goffman reported that a participant could use the occasion to influence other participants by dramatizing the situation. This case of using a situation could be seen in the commentary by XY/C.82.S, when he accepted that 'I have crapped on those that helped me'; 'it was the stigma I had in the past'; 'I pretended I can facilitate this group, that group'. The student knew that the rules had been broken. When this was pointed out, his reply was, 'I do not know whether it was wisdom or fear'; 'I have to travel'.

These words were dramatically put together, realigned in some cases. Such dramatic behaviour could influence the group culture, the pan-handlers collecting attention to exploit the communicative channel within the group. XY/C.82.S knew the limits and elasticity of the group order after all: having been a 'psychic' patient and now a student nurse, one should be aware of the stigma and the journey.

Those players who knew the elasticity of the group knew that words have weight. Knowing the weight they carried, the players uttered them. These players had done their work before moving on to the scene; they borrowed words such as trust, respect and commitment, playing them back in the same space from which they had taken them, providing a 'cloaked safety' as XZ/C.82.S pointed out. 'We destroyed the situations you created', stated XH/C.82.S; 'we revelled in the situation', exclaimed KG/C.82S; 'I don't trust this place any more', claimed PL/M87. 'This group is not as it was', exclaimed NO/M88, and JO/Oct88 presented the drama of her experience in training to the group.

These players could occupy a space that would silence any new gambler on the scene. They employed such words as coinage, 'psychological coinage', and played them back on to the same table. Thus, a pretender who learned the game from outside could destroy what had been created, and the partners in the group did not hesitate to make use of the situation (Goffman 1976, 136).

These situations could lead to misrepresentation in the group (Goffman 1953, 66–70), breaking it into regions each with its specific roles: 'this group is not as it was' (NS/M88 commentaries); 'we gain support outside the group from individuals'. Within the activities in the different regions, one could still see a glimpse of authenticity (Goffman 1959, 75–116).

A review of relevant research

What does some of the recent research literature tell us about theory and practice?

Norlan's (1993) work was on the history of mental health nursing, his research being involved with how psychiatric nursing has travelled to where it now is since its conception in 1891. His account covered the age of the Enlightenment up to the present time. The research involved interviewing trained staff and students who had just started the Project 2000 syllabus.

Norlan produced a descriptive account of the role of psychiatric nurses, but he failed to consider the conflicts of role on the part of the students. He made it clear that his thesis approached the situation from an historical perspective, its purpose being only to describe psychiatric nursing from the point of view of the nurse and not to be philosophical or to critique mental health history.

Norlan's recommendation was that patients should be involved in their care. He perceived the move to higher education as one that was good for nursing. We could say that Batty (1703–76) wanted his attendants to come from the 'gentle' class, but now that we have achieved Batty's wish with the attendants bred by the Butler education system, the health service and the health-care trusts, will they make any change to the process of attending? Norlan also recommended that more research be undertaken on historical perspectives. He perceived that the case management approach to care, the key-worker system, in operation in USA, could be of use to British nurses.

The current project moved beyond the Enlightenment, presenting a transcultural view of madness and its management. It also draws the categories for presenting the students' lived experience from history and presents a philosophy for mental health nursing. What would have been of interest is to compare the perception of caring from Norlan's work with the experience of training of the students involved in this research. Such a project is, however, beyond the remit of this work. The work of Porter (1985) went back as far as Greek times to show that the principle of care has not altered greatly and that madness was in ancient times regarded as curable.

Towell's (1975) project was concerned with the socialization of mental health nurses, both in and out of work. He took an ethnographic approach, moving into the nurses' residences and spending a lot of time on the ward. Towell's thesis described what the student nurses did during their three years of training. In the student accounts presented in the current thesis, the data dealt with the social, economic and, in some cases, family issues of the students. It gave an account of the social life of students in and out of work and how being a nurse influenced their level of social interaction. Although the two projects have approached the topic from different angles, Towell's dealing with socialization and mine considering the use of experience in training, both showed aspects of the social life of mental health student nurses.

Morrison's (1994) thesis dealt with exploring care from the patients' perspective of how they viewed the nursing staff (qualified nurses). The patients involved were not psychiatric clients, nor were the nursing staff trained mental health nurses. Morrison pointed out the 'power issue' between the nurses and patients, although he found evidence of a commitment to caring. Morrison recommended that patients should be encouraged to be involved in their care.

In my thesis, the mental health nurse students seemed to be pragmatic in how they played their role, the issue of power and control between them and the client not being particularly stressed. The students in my sample perceived the work situation to be a kind of tension and friction that might or might not be confronted. They saw their clients/patients as their source of knowledge, people from whom they learned. They displayed much concern for those in their care and made it obvious that their main concern and responsibility lay towards their patients.

Lathlean's (1995) research was concerned with the implementation and development of the lecturer practitioner role in nursing. Classroom teaching was seen as a decontextualized situation, and practice was seen as caring for patients as a member of the workforce and learning whilst doing. The project involved investigating the role of the ward sister or ward manager as a lecturer practitioner, someone linking learning and practice. These lecturer practitioners described their role as ward work and university work. The function of the lecturer practitioner was to reflect on clinical situations with a group of students.

The technique used was based on the work of Schön (1983). This approach has its problems as some students in the current project have pointed out that reflection can involve transference and projection from one clinical situation to another. The question at issue for the students was not so much the relationship between practice and theory but knowing the theory and the patient and being aware of how to practise. Newman (1997), in his extensive work on Schön, from the man, the philosopher to lecturer practitioner, has subjected Schön's philosophy to a detailed critique. Papell and Skolnik (1992), in a critique of Schön's philosophy in relation to social workers, pointed out that there is no ethical standpoint in terms of different cultural peculiarities in Schön's work.

The theory–practice gap seemed to be an issue in my research, some students making the point that school activity could not bridge the gap, others seeing theory and practice as an embodiment involving knowledge, skills, an ethical dimension of action and support. Some students believed that the gap could be bridged by the help of the supervisor. The best way to learn was 'get in', 'do it and then go over it with the supervisor'. Others stated that 'do your research, know your patient and you are respected' in practice. The point the students make about the support group questioning the clinical situations with students at different levels of training showed that they were undertaking the task of bridging the gap. The presence of a lecturer, as requested by the group, might also have been of great use.

My own research, together with the recent literature, shows the difficulty of students being able to reflect systematically upon their own experience. If the notion of reflective practice is to be meaningful, it is clear that institutions need to provide the appropriate structures within which it can develop, and students themselves need the opportunity sometimes to be able to confront the self-deceptions that are readily to hand.

Developing a philosophy for mental health care with a developmental approach towards reflective practice

Above, we considered the data and how they could be interpreted, the literature search including the comments and observations of the students. This next part will deal with personal knowledge and its relation to practice under the following headings:

- Personal knowledge
- Reflection-on-experience
- A form of experiential learning
- A developmental approach to reflective practice

Personal knowledge

MacMurray (1953–54), in *Persons in Relation*, distinguishes two modes of our knowledge of other people, which might be termed 'objective' and 'subjective'. He gives the example of a teacher of psychology who is visited by a pupil wishing to consult him about his work. The interview begins as a simple personal conversation between them, but during its course, it becomes clear that there is something wrong with the pupil. The psychologist becomes aware that the pupil's behaviour is hysterical. As a result, his attitude towards him changes from a personal to an impersonal one; he adopts an objective attitude, and the pupil takes on the character of an object to be studied. This new attitude of the teacher towards the pupil is abnormal from the point of view of the relationship between teacher and pupil, but it is the normal attitude of a psychologist pursuing research into behaviour. It is, in fact, an attitude that makes any activity scientific.

Thus the relationship of one person to another may either be personal or impersonal. Personal knowledge assumes that men are free agents, responsible for their behaviour and acting in accordance with the distinction between right and wrong; impersonal knowledge assumes that all human behaviour follows determined patterns and that the laws obeyed by behaviour are discoverable by objective, scientific methods of investigation. It is conventionally asserted that, of these two incompatible forms of knowledge, the objective one must be true, since we assume that what is objective is true and what is subjective is false.

MacMurray thinks that it is an emotional prejudice that is responsible for this view. The term 'objective' does not mean 'true', for objective statements are often false. Nor is the term 'scientific' synonymous with correct, for many scientific theories have been abandoned as being incorrect. 'If our generation tends to associate truth with science and objectivity, the association rests upon no logical implication, but only on an emotional prejudice in favour of science' (MacMurray 1961, 31). Any personal activity, including science, must have a motive, and all motives are in an important sense emotional. The scientific state of mind is therefore one kind of emotional state rather than a motiveless pursuit.

MacMurray believes the personal and impersonal attitudes to be complementary, the personal being the more fundamental. If one person treats another impersonally, he treats him as if he were an object rather than a person, negating the personal character of the other. 'The impersonal attitude in a personal relation is the negative which is necessarily included in the positive personal attitude, and without which it could not exist' (MacMurray 1961, 34).

Even in the most personal of relationships, the other person is in fact an object for us as we see his movements and so on but do not perceive these as mere movements. We apprehend through them the intentions, thoughts and feelings of the other. In the language of Gestalt theory, the movements are the ground against which we perceive the person as person, or as Polanyi (1958) would put it, the impersonal is apprehended tacitly, the personal explicitly. Thus, the impersonal aspect of the personal relation is always present. MacMurray says that, in a personal relationship between persons, an impersonal relationship is necessarily included and subordinated. The negative occurs for the sake of the positive.

An impersonal relation, however, reverses this. The personal is subordinated to the impersonal, as in slavery. In such a relationship, the negative dominates the positive as the personal qualities of the slave are subordinated to the master's own impersonal intention. Now, a personal relationship requires no justification, being its own end, but an impersonal relationship always requires justification: we have to ask of any impersonal attitude (e.g. science or slavery) under what conditions it is justifiable, whereas this question appears absurd with regard to the personal attitude. MacMurray believes that the proper answer to this question is that the impersonal attitude is justifiable when it is itself subordinated to the personal attitude.

There are, then, two types of knowledge – a knowledge of persons as persons and a knowledge of persons as objects. When we reflect upon these, two specific types of intellectual activity arise. When the attitude is personal, this reflective activity will be philosophical; in the case of the impersonal, it will be scientific. The question of which is right, the personal conception of man as a free agent or the scientific conception of man as a determined being, arises through a misunderstanding. *Both* are correct because they do not refer to the same field, but this is only the case because the scientific knowledge of man is included and subordinated, as a negative aspect, in the philosophical knowledge of the personal. Philosophical knowledge of persons is the 'full and inclusive knowledge of the personal other, for to be an agent a person must also be a continent object in the world' (MacMurray 1961, 41). Scientific knowledge, on the other hand, is limited and abstract:

> There is then no necessary contradiction between personal freedom and scientific determination in the anthropological field. The 'I do' is indubitable, and to assert it is to assert my freedom as an agent. But when I do this I make no preposterous claim that I can do anything and everything at will and unconditionally. Every actual action is conditioned, both by the determinate nature of the world in which it must be done and by my own determinate nature as an object in that world. Without this determination I could not act at all and so could have no freedom. If then I abstract this determinate aspect of action by limitation of attention, and seek to understand it, the scientific method is the correct one, and the only possible one. (MacMurray 1961, 41)

If, however, I believe the scientific view to be the only possible view that can be correct, I am in error for this would then be to deny the possibility of the personal attitude that produces it. The 'I' can never depersonalize itself.

The theory/practice issue is a form of dualism that has influenced mental health nursing for a long time and has culminated in a critical situation since the second part of the twentieth century as we can judge from the difficulties the students experienced. The moving of qualified staff from the ward to the classroom and from the classroom to the ward may help to overcome these difficulties, but without a coherent philosophy and set of practices, the dualism may remain.

The type of knowledge on which nurses rely in caring is empirical, deriving from the observations of patients at a clinical level as well as from the empirical sciences of sociology, psychology, biology, nursing and medicine. Nursing is, in a sense, the link agent in the field of care, since it is the personal act of caring that brings together the different regional decisions of other professionals. Sometimes, as the students pointed out, the other disciplines of these regions may choose to retain their knowledge and refuse to share their perspective or justification for it. This creates a kind of power friction and can culminate in students being left with the feeling that they could have benefited from these groups.

The main point is, however, that nursing, as the link agent of care, has to take into account the impersonal information of the medical model and integrate it into the personal knowledge that arises in the day-to-day activity of caring and sharing the patient's life.

This empirical knowing shows itself in both the classroom and the clinic. The students gained from the discussions and project work, and learned how to assert themselves in other situations. The other sources of this empirical knowledge were other people, including medical staff, other students, nursing staff and patients. Thus, the empirical knowing of the students can be seen as having two 'compartments': one knowledge from texts and the other interactive knowing. This type of knowing could be seen as subjective (being mine), objective (emanating from the others) and interactive. It could be said that this form is intersubjectivity/objectivity/situational.

This caring field also displayed another aspect of knowing, caring that forms part of the process that is knowing oneself, that is, the personal experiences not necessarily accessible to others. This is the type of knowing that the students referred to as their 'own yardstick of self-measurement'. This type of knowing through reflection and awareness is that of personal development. Addressing this issue will lead us to a developmental, reflective approach to caring/self-care.

These two aspects of knowing – knowing the professional concepts of work events and knowing in terms of self-development – are both embodied in our actions and are both possibilities of openness. However, as was pointed out earlier, self-knowledge is not an automatic process: it requires its own discipline and may be hindered by the tensions of the workplace. Trainee nurses, as other human beings, bring their own history to the task of caring for others, and the programme designed here to encourage learning through reflection-on-experience must have this taken into account.

Reflection-on-experience

The space in which the students developed their skills is, as we have seen, described as 'being thrown in the deep end', but, as Merleau-Ponty has argued, to be thrown is not to be devoid of history but to be in the centre of objectivity and subjectivity; it is 'a distance from my past with all its fortuitous events, a definite significance', and by pursuing with a future plan one will find out how that plan 'had been foreshadowed by it', thus introducing historicity into one's life (Merleau-Ponty 1962, 346).

In a very real sense, we discover our histories only by further acts of commitment revealing how we are determined by our past, but these same acts allow us to carry forward our past into a future. This act of carrying forward is thus both the grounding of and the impediment to the rationality of my person and history.

This influence of the passage of time on the students could be seen in category 1, subcategory c, in which the students described how their educational experiences in the past still influenced their plan. In category 4, subcategory b, some found that their past style of education was too directive, and they still called for direction. Others felt that the style to which they were exposed enhanced self-directed learning, and they wanted a plan of training to develop their own study.

Past personal experiences were described by the students during group discussion in the classroom. HT/C.82.S described the experience as, 'my whole life opened up in front of me; I have just left the house I was born in, the discussion brings back my 28 years'. The discussion that started in the classroom carried on outside in the students' own life. A dialogue with someone who was caring and supportive was the form of confronting and transcending the situation. In conversation, our perspectives of life merge into each other, and we co-exist through a common world. 'In the experience of dialogue, there is constituted between the other person and myself a common ground, my thoughts and his are interwoven into a single fabric' (Merleau-Ponty 1962, 354).

The discussion is a shared operation for each other, and we co-exist through a common world. Especially valuable is this form of reciprocity with trust in the anticipated response of the others. It was this 'trust which created care' (HT/C.82.S, category 6, subcategory d). This anticipated response is faith in what we can expect in a situation. Action is faith built on trust, a form of communion with the world (Merleau-Ponty 1962).

This world is shared with others. We are not empirical beings or merely 'automatons'. JX/C.82.S says, 'it involved what I am' and 'I am valued for what I do'; 'It is my personal development, the moment I realized that it is not the case, I won't be doing psychiatric nursing.'

In these situations, I must be aware of 'my own projection' (JX/C.82.S). My experience might be similar to, but not the same as, that of others. In dealing with the other, 'I learn' while 'being on the job'. Through dialogue with the patients, the students confront their own lived experiences and at the same time assist the patients. Whilst talking with the patient, 'my whole life enfolds', 'it's like reliving the past' and 'I came out having learnt more about myself'. This was how the students described learning experiences when being thrown in: 'you just do it', 'talk to the patient', and then reflect on it with your supervisor with a theoretical perspective. 'This is how we learned' (see the M88 commentaries in Ramsamy 1998 and category 1, subcategories a and c). It was through dialogue and social encounter with the patients (see Ramsamy 1998, 234–7) that they confronted themselves and in the process helped the patients. 'You know you have been of some help when they come and thank you' (see the M88 commentaries in Ramsamy 1998).

This shared world in which our 'blood flows' is a system of experience in which 'we communicate'. The world is the field of all the fields. What appears in one field of experience provides a 'primordial setting in relation to the world' (Merleau-Ponty 1962, 351). The shared field of the School 'takes us to the ward situations', and 'the ward situations take me back to the School group discussion'.

Students found that what they learned through their work with patients was self-development for their experiences: 'it helps you to express yourself during ward rounds and case conferences'; 'It gives you confidence'; 'you are respected'. In such situations, they grasp the visibility of their own personal development with their development as professionals. This is the power of the self, the power to move and create the synthesis between what is seen and what is personal. In this case, the practice is not a form of automation, nor is it knowing a kind of theory simply to apply it; instead, it is the embodiment of a power that can be directed by reflection.

Reflection occurs in action and on action and could be seen in the case where the students used their own life experiences to reflect upon their work, their project, then using this learning experience in clinical situations, and subsequently reflecting on the whole issue during discussion in the classroom. This approach to learning had been well documented by Schön (1983) and Polanyi (1966).

In situations in which the students were involved in dialogue with the patients using their own pre-reflective experiences to focus on the close proximity of the patients' situations, they did so with trust in the 'arm band'. They had faith in the power of the 'arm band' as this allowed them to inhabit the shared world of the caring field. In relation to this caring field, argued Heidegger (1978, 439–41):

> Caring understands itself in terms of that which it encounters in the environment and that with which it is circumspectively concerned. This

understanding is not just a bare taking cognizance of itself, such as accompanies all ways of caring. Understanding signifies one's projecting oneself upon one's current possibilities of being-in-the-world, that is to say, it signifies existence as this possibilities. Thus understanding a common sense constitutes even the inauthentic existence of the 'thing'. When we are with one another in public, our everyday concern does not encounter what is 'given' along with these 'affairs, undertakings, incidents, mishaps'. The words belong to everyday trade and traffic as the soil from which they grow and the arena where they are displayed. When we are with one another in public, the others are encountered in activities of such a kind that one is 'in the swim' with it 'oneself'. One is acquainted with it, discusses it, encourages it, combats it, retains it and forgets it, but one always does so primarily with regard to what is getting done and what is 'going to come of it'. We compute the progress which the individual Dasein has made, his stoppages, re-adjustments and output; and we do so proximally in terms of that with which 'he' is concerned – its course, its status, its changes, its availability. No matter how trivial it may be to allude to the way in which Dasein is understood in everyday common sense. Ontologically this understanding is by no means transparent in terms of what it is concerned with, and what it experiences is the 'connectedness' with what Dasein dwells alongside with belongs to history too, not just the isolated running off of 'streams of experience' in individual subjects. Dasein exists factically, it already encounters that which has been discovered within the world. With the existence of historical being-in-the-world, what is ready-to-hand and what is present at hand, have already in every case been incorporated into the history of the world.

In the above discussion, we have seen that the caring of the mental health nurse involves the embodiment of experience in which empirical knowledge and personal knowledge are the flesh and blood. We are in the world and share our time and space with others, and as such, we are acting as agents for each other. Next, using the reported student experiences, I will describe a form of experiential learning used by the groups that I taught. This will be followed by a developmental approach to reflection.

A form of experiential learning

The students described the style of learning to which they were exposed. XJ/C.82.S described the start of the course as being a broad discussion group in which students shared their experiences. According to XZ/C.82.S, the discussion turned into a kind of group therapy in which there was no prescription of how to deal with the issues to which they were exposed. This group discussion and sharing of feelings made CC/C.82.S. feel as if it were close to forming relationships with patients and feel worried about it.

UB/C.82.S. said that there was an initial broad-based discussion, which set the theme for the start of the course, and from then on the course developed by questioning what should be done to meet the needs of the course and clinical requirements. The course was seen as being built from experiences to meet society's needs.

XZ/C.82.S. felt that there was 'cloaked safety' but RK/C.82S felt hurt through breach of confidentiality. HT/C.82.S. felt that there was respect and trust in the group, whereas XY/C.82.S. felt that the journey had to be made even though it meant breaking the rules of trust and safety.

The sharing of personal experiences appeared to help the students to develop as persons and assert themselves in clinical situations. From these accounts, I will describe how the group evolved and developed from 1987, and I will use recent literature to describe the form that this experiential learning took.

The teaching style started from the experiences of the students and the group tutors/lecturers. Heron (1996, 78–9) clarified that this style of teaching should start with 'culture-setting', which means outlining the rules and regulations under which learning will take place. In nursing, since the purpose is to train a professional person, the rules and regulations of the course should be included. They should also comprise the rules of the professional body, the Act of Parliament controlling care, and what is expected from the participants on the course in relation to what the ENB and the university demand from them as students. In addition, health authority requirements should be acknowledged as the students' practice will be based upon their sedimented knowledge and experience in action.

Taking these conditions into account, broad discussions based on the lived experiences of the participants could be described. The description could incorporate the experiences of others in relation to them (Heron 1996, Smyth 1996, Tisdell 1996) as well as covering autobiography or the biography of others.

These discussions or case studies will provide the members and the facilitator with the information for developing 'the discussion theme building' (Tisdell 1996). Heron (1996) makes the point that the discussion theme for developing this style of teaching should be the responsibility of the facilitator, meaning that the facilitator should retain the decision over how the training programme should develop. The facilitator should have the unilateral decision of planning and be able to add what is needed to meet the course requirements. In a sense, the facilitator gives the course a structure, the contents being built from the discussions and the conditions for sharing experiences and knowledge. It is these conditions which direct the process of training.

After the theme-building has been given a clear structure, students' concerns are then collected to form the checklist for discussion. The discussion could then take the form of project work, largely self-directed and allowing the course members to relate to their own experiences. Self-direction in this sense requires direction from the facilitator in that the work produced is supervised and guidance is given on how to improve the standard and quality of the projects.

In the presentations, the members confront their experiences in relation to texts that they have chosen. This style of confronting is what will influence their life experiences in that the search for meaning and the willingness to learn can affect the students at a personal level. The confrontation could take into account the cultural, political and ethical dimension of inquiry. Learning in this form is the embodiment of lived experiences in relation with others, reflection being the cutting edge of reconstructing or deconstructing experiential self-embodiment.

This approach encourages students to get involved in research techniques and activities. Through the process of self-confronting in their search for meaning, they arranged their personal style of being with others, and it is this knowing and being with others during their work that enhanced their personal confidence and development of self. It is this style and support which will influence assertiveness in practice (see category 2, subcategories a and b).

Once the checklist created by the group has been covered, other issues relevant to the clinical needs can be added by the students, based on their clinical experiences, or by the facilitator, thus taking a developmental approach that could also include the future needs of caring. This process is seen in the summaries by UG/C.82.S. (see category 1, subcategory a in Ramsamy 1998).

This approach, it could be argued, is a problem since the facilitator decides the themes, and their arrangement could hamper creativity and autonomy. However, we need to examine here the conditions under which creativity and autonomy can develop. Self-development requires structure and tradition. As Musil points out, what tradition hands down 'is not decades but millenniums' and 'even the spontaneity of an artist is inconceivable without handed down forms and concepts: it is those very handed down forms that become a source of originality' (1978, 1250).

Hauser (1951) insisted that conventional forms of expression themselves help to create the content of what is to be expressed. Hence even though it is true that 'expression always moves on well-worn tracks, they multiply and bifurcate as they are being travelled' (Musil 1951, 21). Wittgenstein expressed such a view when he says that if every composer changed the rules but the variation was very slight, not all the rules being changed, 'the music was still good by a great many of the old rules' (Wittgenstein 1967, 6). As Merleau-Ponty (1962) puts it, it is this sediment of tradition that gives us faith in our action of embracing and in being in communion with the world. It is as if traditions are written into our muscles, the very part of our flesh (Merleau-Ponty 1965).

Manger (1883) saw it as a form of subconscious, wisdom manifested in the institution at an organic level, and warned the reshapers of society. Von Hayek (1979) stressed that once we owe the order of our society to a tradition of rules, which we only imperfectly understand, all progress must be based on tradition.

A developmental approach to reflective practice

This thesis has itself been a process of reflection upon the history of psychiatric care and upon students' experiences. The historical accounts showed how reflection was a powerful tool in the Vedic time in preparing the fighter to face his mentor in defending the nation. The power of reflection was the domain of the god, Braham knowledge being in control. The Egyptians refined their tools for curing madness, moving from the technique of managing the environment to that of attempting to cure madness. Socrates stressed the importance of cognitive control, and the republic was to have citizens at different levels of refinement, depending on the abilities and skills displayed.

The point that reflection occurs at different levels can be seen in the students' accounts (category 5, subcategory c), where they made the point that the level of responsibility they were given depended on their stage of training – least in the first year of training, although in the third year 'they were expected to be in charge'. In category 5, subcategory a, some of the students commented that the other professionals in the caring field were at a different level of knowledge and skill compared with them. 'Knowing your patient and doing your research' were seen as what enhanced one's situation, so there was nothing as practical as a good theory, and this was what the students asked for: 'we want to be taught', 'we want direction' (M88; see Ramsamy 1998).

Above, we saw how learning is embodied in the personal histories of those who care for patients. We have also seen that learning is best facilitated in an environment in which there is dialectical tension between immediate concrete situations (clinical and personal experiences) and analytical detachment (peer support group and reflection on practice). The direction of movement at the crossroads of decision-making during the dialogue between the students and the patients was left to their personal experiences and their power of reflection in practice. This involved knowing the patient; as Charcot informed Freud during a discussion, 'La théorie c'est bien mais ca n'empêche d'exister' (It is a good thing to be concerned about theory, but now knowing it does not affect my existence)(see Lewis 1981, 6). Charcot was concerned about a descriptive approach to the patient's situation rather than about the basic unit of human experiences. It was through a dialogue with the patient that the students assisted in care and at the same time confronted themselves.

Reflection is therefore not a passive process but involves gathering resources or sustenance to fire awareness; as Heraclitus stated, knowledge is formed from a friction of opposites during dialectical tensions. Dewey (1933) argued for reflective activity, stating that there are different levels of knowing. Boud, Keogh and Walken (1985) put a case for experiences to be viewed in stages in relation to learning.

The students' accounts (category 1, subcategory a, UG/C.82.S) showed that negotiation in the planning of training on the part of students could be practised, or had been practised, by reflecting on what had been done and by considering future plans. I will base my own developmental approach to reflection on Kierkegaard's (1945) stages on life's way, taking into account what the students had to say during their conversations. This model has been advanced by Handal and Lauvas (1987), based on the work of Lovlie (1974).

These authors put forward three levels of promoting reflection for student teachers; I have applied their model and developed a fourth level to meet the needs of mental health nurses. The levels are:

- first level – manifest action;
- second level – planning and reflection;
- third level – ethical consideration;
- fourth level – autonomy in practice.

All the stages should take into account the ethical dimension of care during interaction as this dimension is what informs the source of dialectical tension and can prevent conflict developing. At the third level – ethical consideration – this should include not only the ethics of personal and existential experiences, but also the political and the historical dimension of the individual as well as the ethical approach of care being considered. The four levels are described below.

First level: manifest action

This involves finding out the basic rules and regulations concerning human interaction, followed by discussions on how these conditions operate in the relationship between nurse and patient.

Developing a model of case study

Here information relating to the patient is presented. This can take the form of an account of the life events of the patients and what brought them into contact with the mental health care services. This latter consists of teasing out the main events in the patient's life that will be used in the caring intervention. The account should be descriptive, in writing, detailing the interaction with the carer, the patient's biography and the personal experience of the student in relation to the patient.

Second level: planning and reflection

This involves presenting the information to the supervisor (lecturer or clinician) in discussion form, other students on the placement taking part. This will display the different levels at which each student is working – the dialectical tension in the caring field. The next move is the analytical detachment, which involves placing the personal experiential account into a theoretical framework and deciding on the approach of care that may be followed. A documentation of the discussion and referencing the work in terms of theoretical sources could act as a journal of learning.

Third level: ethical consideration

This involves a reflection on other possible modes of care intervention with the lecturer/supervisor. The discussion should be backed by references to the theoretical frameworks of caring approaches. This includes questioning the moral ethical and political aspects of care and challenging and confronting one's personal application to practice. At this level, there develops the ability to operate in a clinical situation using personal knowledge, and this involves caring for oneself and others.

Fourth level: autonomy in practice

Formally defined, autonomy is the capacity to make independent, rationally and morally grounded decisions. As 'existing individuals', in Kierkegaard's (1846) sense, we have the obligation to take responsibility for our own decisions; at the highest level of existence, this necessarily entails a commitment through acts ('leaps') of faith. This is based on sedimented experience, acting with intuition and the ability to make instant decisions, communing with the world with faith – openness in practice. Kierkegaard (1846, 176) stated that 'we are all of us existing individual'. Each individual is responsible for his or her own actions during existence, and our decisions are taken in solitude.

But this decision-making is not that of a solitary individual since we are engaged in particular situations. We are always in a position in which we need to enter into a dialogue with others and share our 'embodied' actions through perception and caring. Autonomy is not absolute but 'embodied' or 'incarnated' (Merleau-Ponty 1962). We have the power to do things only within a social space and not out of our own making or choosing (Spurling 1977, 119). We are not free to do as we please. To achieve autonomy is a task we have to work at and devote ourselves to. As Polanyi (1958) has argued, scientists have to learn their trade from the masters. This involves respect, commitment and responsibility in their situation. It is this place into which they pour their passion in order to bring about innovation and change. Any new members have to learn the established rules and skills.

Autonomy then is passion, knowledge, feeling and the 'embodied perception' that is poured into the situation. Autonomy is grounded in our skills and knowledge but is itself the necessary ground of freedom. It is by 'becoming involved in the world, through stable organs and pre-established circuits that we can acquire mental and practical space which will theoretically free us from our environment and allow us to see it' (Merleau-Ponty 1962, 87).

To become a psychiatric nurse does not mean using my past experience to do as I want: it involves entering into dialogue with clients and other care professionals who are involved in the same situation. The situation has established circuits and habits that are entrenched. My power and autonomy can only develop by my commitment to the situation in which I find myself.

Our actions have a direction: they are always directed towards something; they are intentional. If I act in a specific way in a situation, it is because I have faith in it. There is always order and intelligibility in the world, but this does not mean that it is because it is determined or predestined. The reason is that we intentionally structure our world, and through our concerted actions in the world, we institute social rules and patterns and cannons of intelligibility (Spurling 1977, 120). Autonomy is not an unconstrained act of the will but a quality of all actions, whether or not actively realized (Merleau-Ponty 1962, 435–6).

Our autonomy is 'determinate' because 'existence is determinate'. This implies that the capacity to make existential choices for creative enactment is based on the grounds of our sedimented knowledge. Autonomy is synonymous with transcendence, the capacity to go beyond our created sedimented experience, skills or knowledge in order to develop new ways of dealing with our situation. It is the ability to work and shape our world. Autonomy then is the existential power to change our situation by changing its significance. It is 'appropriating a de facto situation by endowing it with a figurative meaning beyond its real one' (Merleau-Ponty 1962, 172).

This legislative power is not played out in isolation as Sartre (1969) or Kierkegaard would have us believe. Instead, it is employed with others in dialogue. Scientists' rules or discourses are not changed overnight. Change involves much dialogue, passion and time, by which a community commits itself. It is in this way that the real meaning of the situations in which we participate is effectively challenged (Polanyi, 1958, 161–4).

As Polanyi (1958) has argued, it takes time, passion, skills and knowledge from a master to train a doctor. Thus, entering a trade or introducing change is a gradual process demanding commitment in that we have to give our full attention, time and respect to the situation. It is an intentional act directed towards that specific task, which helps us to create the situation. This is not a decision taken by a solitary mental process or via a transient fit of the imagination and then cleared off that then disappears in the next instant. The potentiality for autonomy or transcendence can never 'be extinguished since it co-exists with existence' (Spurling 1977, 122). 'The world is already situated but never completely constituted' (Merleau-Ponty 1962, 435).

From the perspective of autonomous individuals, caring is more than an encounter: it is an opportunity for 'personal development' (XH/C.82.S and UG/C.82.S). It involves action and an openness to the situation with an ethico-political moral stance.

The way forward

> Put a man in the wrong atmosphere and nothing will function as it should. He seems unhealthy in every part. Put him back into his proper element and everything will blossom and look healthy. But if he is not in his right element, what then? Well then he just has to make the best of appearing before the world as a cripple? (Wittgenstein 1945, 43)

The world given to us is largely taken for granted and in this sense pre-reflective; it is found in the derelictions, in the forgotten history, amongst the things we deal with without paying them due attention during our passage. This dereliction and its fragments become of value to us when we direct our attention to them.

What has been discussed up to now was always available for us – the concerns of the students and the history of psychiatric care. But such information can only achieve its critical importance for those involved in this profession if it is contained within a justified view of the nature of caring. In this final section I have argued, following MacMurray, for a philosophy of personal knowledge that enables us both to 'be with' patients and to incorporate the impersonal knowledge of the sciences into our understanding.

In the final analysis, the skill demanded of the psychiatric nurse requires both a detachment in analytic ability and an involvement in the life of the patient. This is why the task of being a carer is not a matter of following prescribed rules but of understanding how such rules are mediated by the patient's own projects and failures. There is no finished theory that can be called upon to make the carer's task a matter of routine, but this book and the thesis that underlies it are written in the hope that a fuller understanding of what is involved in 'knowing the patient' can provide a support for the necessarily difficult and often dramatic process of psychiatric care.

The recommendations arising from this work fall into two parts: first, those concerning practice; and second, those relating to future research. Concerning the former, the following are listed below:

- There is a need to signal in advance to students the course structure and philosophy. This could take the form of a document stating what is expected of students at different levels of training and would take into account the level of reciprocal responsibility between student/students, student/clinical requirements and students/ university.
- The mentor/supervisor should take care of the student for the whole of his or her training.
- There should be a closer contact between the lecturers and those involved in the clinical placements. This could take the form of case study presentations by students at the clinical level. This could take into account the stages of training in relation to the stages of the developmental approach to reflective practice described above.
- Student support groups, organized by lecturers, need to be held at the clinical level. These sessions could meet the immediate clinical need of students through a discussion of clinical situations and their relationship to a theoretical perspective of care.
- A developmental approach to reflection, as described above, should be encouraged, with support from clinicians and lecturers.

As far as further research is concerned, there is a need for more detailed historical studies, but perhaps the greatest need is for further qualitative studies, some of which should be longitudinal, allowing the student voice during training to be heard so that teaching and learning can be most effective.

The research reported in this thesis is aimed primarily at curriculum developers and nurse educators and advances the research literature in these areas in three ways:

1. It provides information on how students perceive the lived world of training.
2. It presents an approach to the use of experience in training that uses a developmental approach to reflective practice with the purpose of developing ways in which trainers can make best use of student experience in training.
3. It develops a philosophy for mental health based on a view of the priority of interpersonal relationships in caring.

References

Ackernecht EH (1968)A Short History of Psychiatry (trans. Wolff S). New York: Hafner.

Adams FR (1969)From association to union: Professional Organisation of Asylum Attendants 1869–1919. British Journal of Sociology 20: 11-26.

Aiyar VAK (1983) The Avatar. In Nathan S (Ed.) Symbolism in Hinduism. Bombay: Central Chinmaya Mission Trust.

Akhilananda Swami (1951) Mental Health and Hindu Psychology. Boston, MA: Brandon Press.

Alexander FG, Selesick ST (1967) The History of Psychiatry: An Evaluation of Psychiatry and Practice from Prehistoric Times to the Present. London: Allen & Unwin.

Alfred C (1961) The rise of the God king. In Piggot S (Ed.) The Dawn of Civilisation. London: Thames & Hudson.

Armand A, Maurer CSB (1982) Mediaeval Philosphy. 2nd Edn. Etiene Gilson Series 4. Ontario: Pontifical Institute of Mediaeval Studies.

Ayyar AA, Giriza A (1957) medicine in the Reg Veda period. Indian Journal of History of Medicine 2(85): 33-6.

Barham P (1984) Schizophrenia and Human Values. Oxford: Basil Blackwell.

Barker E (1929) Greek Medicine (trans. Brock AJ) London: Dent & Son.

Barnes J (1987) Early Greek Philosophy: Harmondsworth: Penguin.

Barns CJ (1976) Modern development in psychiatric nursing. In Baker AA Comprehensive Psychiatric Care. Oxford: Blackwell Scientific.

Barton WR (1959) Institutional Neurosis. Bristol: John Wright.

Batty W (1758) A treatise on madness. In Whiston & White, Hunter R, MacAlpine I (1963) The Three Hundred Years of Psychiatry 1535–1860 (A History Presented in Selected English Text). London: Oxford University Press.

Bhaktivedanta Swami, Prabhupanda AC (1986) Bhagavand-Gita as it Is. Germany: Bharkivedanta Book Trust.

Boud D, Keogh R, Walken D (985) Reflection Turning Experience into Learning. London: Kegan Paul.

Carpenter M (1980) Asylum nursing before 1914. A chapter in the history of labour. In Davies C (Ed.) Re-Writing Nursing History. Hampshire: Croom Helm.

Chinmayananda S(1974) Medition and Life. Madras: Chinmayan Publishing Trust.

Chinmayananda S (1978) The Art of Man Marking. Bombay: Saction Offset.

Chinmayananda S (1979) Vedenta, the Science of Life. Understanding Human Nature, Part 1. Bombay: Chinmaya Mission Trust.

Chinmayananda S (1983) Religion and the new man. In Nathan RS Symbolism in Hinduism. Bombay: Central Chinmaya Mission Trust.

Connelly J (1856) On the Treatment of Insanity. London: Dawsons.

Cotgrove S (1967) The Science of Society. London: George Allen & Unwin.

Dewey J (1933) How we Think. Boston, MA: DC Heath.

Edelstein L (1967) Ancient Medicine (trans. Tamkin O, Temkin CC) Baltimore, MD: John Hopkins University Press.

Ellenberger HF(1974) Psychiatry from Ancient to Modern Times. New York: Basic Books.

Foucault M (1961) Madness and Civilisation. London: Tavistock.

Goffman E (1953) Communication Conduct in an Island Community. PhD thesis. Chicago, IL: University of Chicago.

Goffman E (1959) The Presentation of Self in Everyday Life. Harmondsworth: Penguin.

Goffman E (1961) Asylum: Garden City, NY: Doubleday.

Goffman E (1976) Strategic Interaction. Oxford: Basil Blackwell.

Handal G, Lauvas P (1987) Promoting Reflective Teaching: Supervision in Practice. Milton Keynes: Open University Press.

Harris CRS (1973) The Heart and the Vascular System in Ancient Greek Medicine from Alcmaeon to Galen. Oxford: Clarendon Press.

Hauser A (1951) The Sociology of Art. London: Routledge & Kegan Paul.

Hawkes J (1980) Introduction to the Odyssey (trans. Rien EV) Homer - Odyssey, London: Sedgwick & Jackson.

Heidegger M (1978) Being and Time. Oxford: Basil Blackwell.

Heron J (1996) Helping the whole people learn. In Boud D (Ed.) Working with Experience. London: Routledge.

Hood MSF (1961) The home of the heroes. In Piggot S (Ed.) The Dawn of Civilization. London: Thames & Hudson.

Hunter R, MacAlpine I (1963) Three Hundred Years of Psychiatry, 1535–1860 (A History Presented in Selected English Text). London: Oxford University Press.

Husserl E (1969) Formal and Transcendental Logic (trans. Cairns D). The Hague: Nijhoff.

Jones C (1989) The Charitable Imperative, Hospitals and Nursing in Ancient Regime and Revoluntionary France. London: Routledge.

Jones K (1972) A History of the Mental Health Services. London: Routledge & Kegan Paul.

Jones WHS (1946) Philosophy and medicine in Ancient Greece. In Sigerist HE, Miller GS (Eds) Supplements of the Bulletin of the History of Medicine No.8. Baltimore, MD: John Hopkins Press.

Kaplan HI, Sadock BI (1985) Comprehensive Textbook of Psychiatry. Vol. 1. London: Williams & Wilkins.

Kelly GA (1955) The Psychology of Personal Construct. New York: Morton.

Kierkegaard S (1846) Concluding Unscientific Postscript to the Philosophical Fragments. Princeton, NJ: Princeton University Press.

Kierkegaard S (1945) Stages on Life's Way (trans. Lowrie W) Princeton, NJ: Princeton University Press.

Kraepelin E (1962) One Hundred Years of Psychiatry. London: Peter Owen.

Laing RD (1960) The Divided Self. London: Tavistock.

Laing RD (1976) The Politics of Experience, and The Bird of Paradise. London: Tavistock.

Lathlean J (1995) The Implementation and Development of Lecturer Practitioner Roles in Nursing. London: Ashdale Press.

Lethrer K.(1989) Thomas Reid. London: Routledge.

Lewis HB (1981) Freud and Modern Psychology. Vol. 1. The Emotional Basis of Mental Illness. New Haven, CT: Yale University.

Lovlie L (1974) Pedagogisk Filosofi for Grakiserance Laerera. Philosophy of Education for Practicing Teachers. Pedagogan 1(22): 19–36.

MacDonald M (1981) Mythical Bedlam: Madness, Anxieties and Healing in Seventeenth Century England. Cambridge: Cambridge University Press.

McGuiness B (1982) Wittgenstein L and his Time. Oxford: Basil Blackwell.

MacMurray J (1953–54) The Self as Agent. London: Faber & Faber.

MacMurray J (1961) Persons in Relation. London: Faber & Faber.

Manger C (1883) Unters Uddchungen Uberdie Methode der Sozialwissenschaften, as reported in Von Hayek FA (Ed.) The Collected Works of Manger C. Vol 2. London: School of Economics.

Maslow A (1968) Towards the Psychology of Being. New York: Van Nostrand Reinhold.

Merleau-Ponty M (1962) Phenomenology of Perception. London: Routledge & Kegan Paul.

Merleau-Ponty M (1965) Structure of Behaviour. London: Methuen.

Mishima Y (1962) Confessions of a Mask (trans. Weatherby M). London: Panther Books.

Morrison P (1994) Understanding Patients. London: Baillière Tindall.

Musil R (1978) Gesammete Werke (Ed. Trise A). Vol.8. Reinbekbei, Hamburg: Rowohlt.

Nathan SR (1983) Ekam Sat Vipa: Bahuda Vedanta. In Nathan SR (Ed.) Symbolism in Hinduism. Bombay: Central Chinmaya Mission Trust.

Newington HH, Bolton JS, Craig M et al (1909) Handbook for Attendants of the Insane. London: Baillière Tindall & Cox.

Newman SJ (1997) Teacher Education and Professional Development: The Work of Donald A. Schön Reconsidered. PhD thesis, University of Sheffield.

Norlan P (1993) A History of Mental Health Nursing. London: Chapman & Hall.

Papell CP, Skolnik L (1992) The reflective practitioner. A contemporary paradigms relevance for social work education. Journal of Social Work Education 28(1): 18-26.

Parry-Jones WF (1972) The Trade of Lunacy: A Study of Private Mad Houses in England in the 18th and 19th Centuries. London: Routledge & Kegan Paul.

Pillau K (1979) History of Cedha Medicine. Tamil Naidu: Government of Tamil Naidu.

Plato (1974) The Republic (trans. Lee D) Harmondsworth: Penguin.

Plomer W (1977) Kilverton's Diary. London: Penguin.

Polanyi M (1958) Personal Knowledge. London: Routledge & Kegan Paul.

Polanyi M (1966) The Tacit Dimension. Garden City, New York: Doubleday.

Porter R (Ed.) (1985) The History of Bethlam. London: Routledge.

Ramprogus V (1995) The Deconstruction of Nursing. Avebury: Ashgate Publication.

Ramsamy S (1989) Concepts of Self and their Implications for Therapy. MEd dissertation, University of Sheffield.

Ramsamy S (1998) Caring for Madness: The Role of Experience in the Training of Mental Health Nurses. PhD thesis, University of Sheffield.

Reede JJ (1983) Universal symbolism. In Nathan SR (Ed.) Symbolism in Hinduism. Bombay: Central Chinmaya Mission Trust.

Ricoeur P (1977) The question of proof in Freud's psychoanalysis writings. Journal of the American Psychoanalytic Association 24(4): 184-210.

Rogers CR (1965) Client-centred Therapy. New York: Houghton Mifflin.

Royal College of Nursing (1942) The Horder Report: The Nursing Reconstruction Committee. London: RCN.

Sartre J (1969) Being and Nothingness. London: Methuen.

Schön D (1983)The Reflective Practitioner. How Professionals Think in Action. New York: Basic Books.

Scull A (1962) Museums of Madness: The Social Organisation of Insanity in Nineteenth Century England. Harmondsworth: Penguin.

Simon B (1978) Mind and Madness in Ancient Greece: The Classical Roots of Modern Psychiatry. London: Cornell University Press.

Smyth J (1996) Developing socially critical educators. In Boud D (Ed.) Working with Experience. London: Routledge.

Spurling L (1977) Phenomenology and the Social World. London: Routledge & Kegan Paul.

Strauss A, Corbin J (1990) Basics of Qualitative Research. Grounded Theory Procedures and Technique. London: Sage.

Szasz T (1961) The Myth of Mental Illness: Foundations of a Theory of Personal Conduct. New York: Harper & Row.

Thorwald J (1962) Science and Secret of Early Medicine (trans. Winston R, Winston C) Cologne: Dumont Press.

Tisdell E (1996) The use of experience to teach feminist theory. In Boud D (Ed.) Working with Experience. London: Routledge.

Towell D (1975) Understanding Psychiatric Nursing. London: RCN.

Tuke DH (1803) Retreat: The State of an Institution Called The Retreat for Persons Afflicted with the Disorders of the Mind. Whitby: Anon.

Von Hayek F (1979) Law, Legislation and Liberty. Vol. 3. London: Routledge & Kegan Paul.

Walker A (1954) Some aspects of the 'moral treatment' of the insane up to 1854. Journal of Mental Health Science 100(421): 807–837.

Weiner DB (1993) The Citizen-Patient in Revolutionary and Imperial Paris. Baltimore, MD: Johns Hopkins University Press.

Wheelan M (1961) Ancient India. In Piggot S (Ed.) The Dawn of Civilization. London: Thames & Hudson.

Whittaker AH (1961) The roots of medical writing (earliest medical texts). Journal of the Michigan State Medical Society, pp 193-9.

Wittgenstein L (1945) Philosophical Investigation (trans. Anscombe GEM). Oxford: Basil Blackwell.

Wittgenstein L (1967) Lectures and Conversation on Aesthetic, Psychology and Religious Beliefs (Ed. Barrett C). Berkeley, CA: University of California Press.

Wood R (1947) The Working Party on the Recruitment and Training of Nurses. London: HMSO.

Zeller E (1963) Outline of the History of Greek Philosophy (trans. Palmer LR) London: Routledge & Kegan Paul.

Index